MINDWEST

— THE LOST BOOK OF —

HERBAL REMEDIES

YOUR **HERBAL APOTHECARY**
FROM **38 HEALING HERBS**

PLANT YOUR **HERB GARDERN**
GROW HERBS OUTDOORS &
CONTAINER GARDENING

Written by SAMANTHA DEERE
Published by LEAFinPRINT

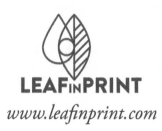

LEAFıₙ**PRINT**
www.leafinprint.com

Midwest–The Lost Book of Herbal Remedies, Unlock the Secrets of Natural Medicine at Home

ISBN: 978-3-907393-25-3

Contents

List of Medical Herbs and Plants

1   Introduction

Step into the enchanting world of plant medicine, where ancient wisdom meets modern healing needs. From the revered traditions of ancient civilizations to the untamed landscapes of the Midwest, herbs are celebrated for their remarkable ability to restore balance, invigorate the body, and nourish the soul. Join me on a captivating journey as we unlock the secrets of the holistic Midwest herbal apothecary, revealing the transformative power of plant medicine in your life.

Imagine a world where vibrant fields of chamomile sway in the gentle breeze, their delicate blooms harboring a soothing remedy for anxious minds. Picture the robust echinacea, standing tall and proud, ready to strengthen your immune system with its potent properties. With the Midwest as your herbal playground, you have the opportunity to cultivate your own healing sanctuary, reaping the benefits of local herbs throughout the seasons.

Holistic healing is more than just a passing trend; it's a profound shift towards embracing nature's innate wisdom. In a society inundated with synthetic medicines and quick fixes, the allure of holistic healing lies in its gentle, natural approach to well-being. It acknowledges the intricate connection between our mind, body, and spirit, emphasizing the importance of nurturing each aspect to achieve true vitality. And at the heart of this transformative journey, we find the extraordinary power of herbs.

This book will empower you to create your own home remedies, offering relief, resilience and nourishment through the seasons. Moreover, in the context of preparedness, discover the ease and assurance that comes with the ability to cultivate and manufacture your medicinal treasures right in the comfort of your own backyard or balcony. This sets the base to embark on a path of holistic well-being and self-sufficiency.

This is what awaits you in this book:

- In the first two chapters (chapters 2 and 3) we set the base for understanding plant medicine in the context of the Midwest. We remind you of what herbal medicine can do for you, what it can't do, and when it is worth consulting an herbalist or allopathic doctor. I also explain the terms used to describe the actions of herbs throughout the book. This vocabulary is essential to understand what effect plants have on our body and mind.

- The next part of this book (chapters 4 and 5) looks at 38 local plants' medicinal properties and where you can source them from. You can buy any plant presented in this book or even directly buy the remedy, I provide you with a step-to-step guide on how to grow herbs outdoors or in containers. This is an opportunity to discover the joy of cultivating your own herb garden, where nature becomes your partner in healing. I will also look at how to store herbs to preserve their aroma and healing properties. However, to develop a relation to your plants and their healing properties, I encourage you to grow at least part of the plants presented here yourself. In the plant description part, many plants have the comment to use its 'recommended dosage' so what is it? For this, please look at Chapter 7.1 Learning About Herbal Dosages.

- The entire second half of this book is dedicated to planning and manufacturing your apothecary table (chapters 6 to 8). It covers topics such as the tools and techniques for making your own herbal medicine, necessary supplies for preparing herbal formulas, techniques to harness the power of herbs, and guidelines for using remedies including herbal dosages, self-monitoring, and when to seek medical support. The suggested remedies are categorized based on specific ailments, and there's also a first-aid herbal remedy kit that provides guidance on which plants to have readily available (on hand) so you can prepare these remedies whenever needed.

- To conclude this book, there is a table that offers an overview of ailments and the herbs that are suitable for preventing and/or treating these conditions (Chapter 9).

2 The Role of Herbalism in Modern Times

2.1 Do I have to choose between Conventional and Herb Medicine?

Conventional medicine has been practiced for approximately 150 years. This timeframe refers to the development and establishment of modern Western medicine as we know it today. It represents the emergence of scientific advancements, standardized medical practices, and the establishment of medical institutions during the 19th century. In contrast, traditional medicine encompasses a range of integrative approaches that have been utilized for thousands of years.

The World Health Organization reports that approximately 80% of the global population relies on herbal medicines as part of their primary healthcare. Therefore, the use of herbs in everyday medicine is commonplace for a significant portion of the world's population. In the Western world, there has been a resurgence of interest in herbal practices in recent years. More people are actively seeking natural alternatives and complementary healthcare approaches. This trend has been steadily growing since the early 2000s, fueled by an increasing awareness of the potential benefits of herbs and a desire for holistic well-being. There has also been a rise in critics of conventional medicine, contributing to the renewed interest in herbal practices.

There is a growing body of scientific research supporting the efficacy and safety of various herbs, further bridging the gap between conventional and herbal medicine. This research is helping to validate the traditional uses of herbs and establish evidence-based practices for their incorporation into modern healthcare.

However, while there is a significant body of scientific research on many herbs and their medicinal properties, it is important to note that not all herbs have been extensively studied or have conclusive scientific evidence to support their claims and uses. One main reason is that conducting thorough studies on herbs presents challenges due to the complexity of herbal formulations. Unlike conventional drugs that often consist of single compounds, herbs contain a diverse array of chemical constituents and interact with the body in complex ways. For example, while aspirin is a simple compound called acetylsalicylic acid, its natural source, white willow bark, contains a more intricate combination of compounds that work together synergistically. This complexity is one of the key advantages of plant-based remedies, as it allows for a broader spectrum of therapeutic effects and potential synergistic interactions between the various compounds present in the herb. But this complexity also makes it difficult to apply the same standardized approach to "proofing" herbal medicine as is done in modern medicine. It requires a nuanced understanding of the unique mechanisms and interactions involved in herbal remedies.

While there is a rich historical and cultural heritage supporting the use of herbs, further research and clinical trials are needed to provide stronger evidence for their efficacy, safety, and potential interactions with conventional medications. This highlights the importance of approaching herbal medicine with an open mind, understanding its limitations, and continuing to encourage scientific exploration to build a more robust foundation of knowledge in this field.

Following this approach, conventional and herbal medicine are not in conflict but can complement each other so you do not have to choose between one and the other. While conventional medicine excels in acute situations, diagnostics, and surgeries, herbal medicine offers a holistic and natural approach to health, prevention, and overall well-being. By integrating both approaches, individuals can benefit from the strengths of each system, achieving a comprehensive and personalized healthcare approach. In an ideal scenario, medicine takes a comprehensive approach, embracing various tools and knowledge to achieve balance, optimize bodily systems, and proactively prevent illnesses. This requires cooperation between different medical perspectives, focusing on the holistic needs of individuals rather than isolated aspects. Surgical procedures and medical interventions play crucial roles, and traditional medicine can provide support by addressing post-surgical pain, managing stress during recovery, and alleviating digestive issues. Traditional healers prioritize the attainment of peace and happiness as fundamental elements of genuine healing. They underscore the significance of having confidence in our interconnectedness and transcending fear and negativity. This confidence is the cornerstone of their approach to healing.

2.2   What Are the Main Precautions to Take When Using Herbs?

When utilizing herbs for medicinal or therapeutic purposes, it is crucial to exercise caution and take necessary precautions. Understanding the main precautions associated with herb usage can help ensure safe and effective outcomes. This section explores key considerations and guidelines to bear in mind when incorporating herbs into your wellness routine.

1. It's important to always monitor yourself for any potential adverse reactions or side effects. While herbs are generally safe and beneficial, individuals may have individual sensitivities or allergies to certain herbs. Pay close attention to how your body responds. Keep track of any changes in your physical or mental well-being and discontinue use if you experience any negative symptoms. It's also advisable to consult with a healthcare professional or herbalist before incorporating new herbs into your routine, especially if you have any pre-existing medical conditions or are taking medications.

2. Herbal medicine may not be free from toxicity and side effects. One has to become aware of what one might feel when taking an herb. One possibility, for instance, is that an herb will initiate a release of toxins from the body. It creates flu-like symptoms. This is known as 'healing crisis' and is a temporary worsening of symptoms that happens after you begin a new alternative medicine treatment. Monitor this reaction as described above.

3. When taking herbs, one must drink water throughout the day. An herb has to move and perform its actions through the water. Think of it this way; Your body is approximately 75% water. When any system has an imbalance, water is required to flush any unwanted substance from the body. Herbs create movement in various systems with the help of water.

4. According to the master herbalist and teacher Michael Tierra, L.AC., O.M.D, one should note that Westerners unfamiliar with herbal medical systems tend to take too little of an herb, conclude that herbs are not effective as a result and discard the treatment. Therefore, please review the dosage section in this book with dosages recommended for each herb carefully.

5. Know the toxicity of an herb, discuss it with a practitioner, and proceed. Awareness and research are the keys. Bear in mind that many herbs can treat a particular issue. There is no reason to use an herb with contraindications if you feel unsafe. Options exist. Well-trained practitioners understand the options and can guide you.

6. Some herbs are more toxic than others. This book avoids those herbs to make the beginner's path more accessible.

7. One must use the right herb for the proper condition. Never think that an herb used to treat asthma will put you to sleep or reduce inflammation. Carefully reading the section describing the different plants (Materia Medica) will allow you to match the herb to the ailment. The table in Chapter 9 represents a summary of the ailments and the herbs suited for each condition presented in this book.

2.3 The Actions of Herbs – Explanation of Action Words

Understanding herbs and their actions is essential. In the previous chapters we covered the differences between conventional medicine and traditional medicine. When the whole herb is used rather than its component, your body responds holistically. You will be amazed at how many things herbs can do. It is truly a wonder.

If you are already taking medication, you must consult with a trustworthy, trained practitioner before taking any herb.

Adaptogens — These help various systems in the body to 'adapt' to stress. Adaptogens protect, restore and strengthen. In many cases, they provide nourishment, just like food. This book includes classic adaptogens: American Ginseng, Tulsi/Holy Basil (*Ocimum sanctum* – not presented in this book) and Elderberry and other herbs with calming and stress-relieving effects: Chamomile, Lavender, Nettle, Roses, Lemon Balm, Rosemary and Sage.

Alterative — Provides nourishment and strength for the body via removing toxic metabolic wastes (often from the liver). This book includes Dandelion, Boneset, Echinacea, Elderberry, Red Clover, Yarrow and Yellow Dock.

Anesthetic — Depresses nerve function, thereby creating a loss of sensation or pain consciousness. This book only deals with topical anesthetics. Examples from this book include Plantain

Anthelmintic — Destroy worms and parasites in the digestive tract. Examples from this book include: Mugwort

Antiemetic — Will reduce nausea and help prevent vomiting. This book includes Meadowsweet and Mint.

Anti-Lithic — These herbs prevent the formation of gravel or stones in the urinary system. An example from this book is Blackberry.

Anti-inflammatory — These work directly on tissues to soothe. They do not interrupt the practical aspects of natural inflammatory reaction, but they reduce the harmful effects of inflammation. This book includes Arnica, Basil, Calendula, California Poppy, Chamomile, Comfrey, Elderberry, Wild Ginger, Goldenrod, Lavender, Lemon Balm, Marshmallow, Meadowsweet, Mint, Mullein, Oregano, Passionflower, Plantain, Roses, Rosemary, Sage, St. John's Wort, Valerian and Yarrow.

Antispasmodic — This eases muscle cramping, as well as muscular tension. Antispasmodics include nervines that reduce psychological and physical stress (the brilliant design of nature!) Some antispasmodics lessen muscle spasms throughout the body, while others work with specific organs or systems. This book includes Black Cohosh, Chamomile, California Poppy, Lemon Balm, Passionflower, Sage, Valerian.

Antitussive — This category prevents coughs, both wet and dry. In this book: Mullein, Passionflower, and Wild Ginger

Antiviral — Prohibits the actions of a virus. This book includes Echinacea, Elderberry, Lemon Balm, St. John's Wort and Wild Ginger.

Astringent — Astringents act to dry out a cell; they squeeze excess fluid from cells and carry unwanted substances out of the body. Astringents bind to mucous membranes. Mucous membranes are the carriers of bacteria and the seeds of illness. Astringents also break up fats and tighten tissues, releasing toxins and thereby improve the quality of fatty impure skin. They assist with weight loss. They help break down proteins, reduce irritation and inflammation, and decrease fluid loss through excessive sweating, vomiting, urination and diarrhea. Examples in this book include Blackberry leaves, Boneset, Calendula, Comfrey, Goldenrod Horsetail, Meadowsweet, Mullein, Plantain, Rosehips, Sage and Yarrow

Bitter (herbs) — These are exceptional herbs that have profound benefits. A bitter herb sends a message to the gut via the central nervous system. It tells the gut to release digestive hormones that stimulate the appetite, give rise to the flow of digestive juices and then increase bile flow. Consequently, the liver receives the signal to work more effectively with bile to detoxify and repair the gut. This book includes Black Cohosh, Boneset, Calendula, California Poppy, Dandelion, American Ginseng, Goldenrod, Horsetail, Milkweed, Meadowsweet, Mint,

Mugwort, Mullein, Nettle, Oregano, Parsley, Passionflower, Plantain, Red Clover, Rosemary, Sage, St.John's Wort, Valerian and Yarrow

Most dark leafy greens are also bitter. They are medicine in and of themselves. Befriend your bitter herbs wholeheartedly. Even though this category of herbs tastes bitter, remember that they clean the liver. The liver executes over 400 different functions. Three essential functions are blood filtration, metabolic stability, and nutrient synthesis. There is hardly a person who does not need to optimize liver function.

Carminative — Carminatives are rich in aromatic oils. They stimulate proper digestion, soothe irritations along the intestinal wall, reduce inflammation in general, help alleviate gas and promote easy elimination. This book includes Basil, Boneset, Chamomile, Dandelion, Echinacea, Wild Ginger, Lemon Balm, Meadowsweet, Mint, Oregano, Parsley, Rosemary, Sage, Thyme and Valerian.

Cardiotonic — A beneficial herb that increases the strength and tone of the heart. Examples from this book include Elderberry, Wild Ginger, Milkweed, Rose, and Yarrow.

Diaphoretic — Opens channels to detoxify and increase perspiration. In the case of bronchitis or chest tightness, it opens the lungs and initiates detoxification. This book includes Elderberry, Boneset, Goldenrod, Wild Ginger, Lemon Balm, Mint, Mugwort, Roses and Rosemary

Diuretic: Increased production of urine by the kidneys. Diuretics work by stimulating the kidneys to remove excess water and electrolytes from the body, leading to increased urine output. In this book: California Poppy, Parsley, Marshmallow

Emetic — It causes vomiting: Examples from this book include Boneset.

Emmenagogue – Promotes the menstrual discharge. In this book: Parsley and Yarrow.

Emollient — Applied to the skin to protect, soften and soothe. Examples from this book include: Plantain (soothes both internally and externally), Oatstraw (soothes both internally and externally)

Expectorant: An expectorant removes mucous or other unwanted substances. This book includes Basil, Boneset, Chamomile, Wild Ginger, Marshmallow and Thyme.

Febrifuge — This lowers a fever. Examples from this book include Basil, Boneset and Yarrow.

Galactagogue — Increases breast milk flow in nursing mothers. Examples from this book include: Nettle (or its cousin Blessed Thistle), Ginger (or Fenugreek seed if you have it on hand).

(California poppy or a simple tea made from fresh parsley can dry up breast milk — the opposite action.)

Hepatics — Hepatics tone and strengthen the liver and increase bile flow. Examples from this book include Dandelion and Oregano.

Hypotensive — This lowers blood pressure. Examples from this book include Wild Ginger, Passionflower and Yarrow.

Laxatives — Laxatives stimulate bowel movements. Proper elimination is the cornerstone of good health. We should not have to rely on laxatives all the time to optimize digestive function. However, they keep us out of trouble until we address our deeper issues. We should consider all aspects of our diet instead of becoming too reliant on laxatives. This book includes Chamomile, (Boneset), Dandelion, and Dock (Yellow).

Nervines — Nervines tone the nervous system and are restorative. They are either nerve tonics that strengthen and restore, nerve relaxants that ease anxiety in the mind and body, or nerve stimulants that work directly on neural activity. This book includes Chamomile, Sage, Lemon Balm, Rose, St. John's Wort and California Poppy.

Oxytocic — Stimulates uterine contractions and assists in childbirth — Examples from this book include: Black Cohosh, Nettle, Sage, Mugwort, Rosemary, and Yarrow. **(On the other hand, if you do not want to stimulate uterine contractions, avoid these herbs.)**

Rubefacient — Dilates the capillaries and increases circulation in the skin. It draws blood from deeper areas of the body to the skin surface. Examples from this book include Rosemary and Wild Ginger.

Sedative — Calms the nerves. Releases stress and nervousness from the body. This book includes California Poppy, Lavender, Passionflower, Sage and Valerian.

Stimulant — Increases speed of physiological functions. Examples from this book include Ginseng, Ginger, Peppermint, and Rosemary.

Styptic — Stops or reduces external bleeding by containing concentrated astringents. Examples from this book include Yarrow, Plantain, and Cattails.

Tonic herbs — strengthen and revitalize a particular organ system or the entire body. This book includes Blackberries, Wild Ginger, Boneset, Dandelion, Horsetail, Nettle and Rosehips.

Vermifuge — Rids the intestines of worms. Examples from this book include: Mugwort (and as an aside, the simple kitchen herb Garlic)

Vulnerary — Contains properties that heal wounds. This book includes Arnica, Boneset, Calendula, Comfrey, Chamomile, Plantain, Horsetail, Mullein and Yarrow

Knowing how herbs behave helps you understand the herbs you will use and will allow you to use them more confidently.

2.4   The Effects of Taste and Temperature

As you progress in your herbal studies, you'll uncover additional properties of herbs such as temperature and taste. Ancient systems like Ayurveda and Traditional Chinese medicine aligned herbs with individual constitutions, with these insights integrated into Chapter 6 (Materia Medica) for a comprehensive guide for advanced herbalists. To delve deeper into understanding individual constitutional types and the corresponding herbs based on Ayurvedic principles, I recommend my book 'Stress Resilience Workbook with Seasonal Herbal Healing Infusions' (*http://www.leafinprint.com/*).

3 Where to get the Herbs for a Well-Rounded Herbal Collection

3.1 Planning your Apothecary Table

Creating an apothecary table is an exciting and fulfilling endeavor for those interested in herbal medicine. It allows you to cultivate a collection of plants that can be used for various purposes, such as teas, tinctures, salves, and more.

Before embarking on your apothecary table journey, it is crucial to assess your specific needs, abilities and goals. Consider the health concerns you wish to address, the types of remedies you want to create, and the herbs that resonate with your personal preferences. Are you looking to support overall wellness, manage specific conditions, or enhance certain aspects of your well-being?

Once you have identified your needs, it's time to select the plants that align with those needs. A helpful starting point is the table in Chapter 9 that offers an overview of the plants presented in this book and the ailments they are suited for. You can delve deeper into the particulars of each herb by exploring the information provided in Chapter 5.If you want to grow them, consider factors such as the plant's growth requirements and your level of experience in cultivating and harvesting them.

Creating an organized functional working space where you prepare your herbs is vital for efficiency and convenience. Determine a suitable location for your table, ensuring it receives adequate natural light and is easily accessible. Consider the available space and plan accordingly, whether it's a dedicated room, a corner of your kitchen, or a designated outdoor area. Arrange your herbs in a way that allows for easy identification and access. Consider using labels or tags to keep track of each plant's name and properties. Additionally, allocate space for storing your tools, such as mortar and pestle, jars, bottles, and scales.

Develop a routine of observing, tending, and nurturing your plants, allowing yourself to be present and attuned to their needs. This connection can enhance the energetic qualities of the herbs and contribute to the overall effectiveness of the remedies you create.

3.2 Sourcing and Selecting High-Quality Local Herbs

It is important to get good quality herbs to cook and make your remedies. You can get them from various sources:

- Grow herbs in your garden or in pots. The next chapters in this book show you how.

- Forage your herbs. While foraging is not the main aim of this book, many of the herbs described can also be foraged. For more details consider my book: "Foraging Medicinal Herbs and Wild Edible Plants in the Great Lakes Region". There I provide details about foraging in the Upper Midwest and Southern Ontario, to forage effectively medicinal plants and wild edibles. You can find it in our Amazon store:

  https://www.amazon.com/author/leafinprint

  or our website: *www.leafinprint.com.*

- Purchase kitchen herbs from any grocery store or purchase them online. If possible, source local herbs from local growers or your farmer's market.

There are a few guidelines to follow when purchasing herbs. Generally, you will need one to four ounces of an herb for non-commercial use. Four ounces is more appropriate for a larger family.

Always make sure that:

1. You choose a reputable herb company.

2. Your herbs have color. An herb that is not vibrant will not contain maximum healing qualities.

3. Your herbs smell. Many herbs have offensive odors. However, if an herb smells, it contains vitality.

4. They must have a taste. Perhaps the herbs may not always taste great. Many herbs (truthfully the best ones for you) often taste bitter or pungent. Yet the distinctive flavor of the herb is significant. It tells you what qualities of the herb work with which parts of the body. However, this is a more advanced concept that you can explore further in your studies.

Remember that herbal remedies should have a direct result. If it does not work:

- It may not be fresh.

- It may be the wrong herb.

- It may take longer to take effect.

- You may be taking the wrong dosage.

Check with a practitioner to see what is causing the problem.

3.3   Storing and Preserving Herbs

Storing and preserving techniques are essential for maximizing the shelf life and maintaining the quality of herbs. Here are some common techniques:

- Drying: Drying is one of the most popular methods for preserving herbs. Harvest the herbs when they are at their peak, tie them in small bundles, and hang them upside down in a well-ventilated area away from direct sunlight. Once completely dry, store the herbs in airtight containers in a cool, dark place. When herbs are properly dried and stored, their medicinal properties can be maintained for up to one year or even longer.

- Freezing: Freezing herbs helps retain their flavor and aroma. Wash and pat dry the herbs, then chop or leave them whole, depending on your preference. Place them in freezer-safe bags or containers and remove any excess air. Label the containers with the herb name and date before storing them in the freezer. Frozen herbs can retain their medicinal properties for around six months to one year.

- Infused Oils and Vinegars: Infusing herbs in oils or vinegars can enhance their flavor and create versatile ingredients. Place clean, dry herbs in a sterilized jar and cover them with oil or vinegar. Seal the jar tightly and store it in a cool, dark place for several weeks to allow the flavors to infuse. Strain the herbs before using the infused oil or vinegar to prevent the mixture from becoming rancid. Infused oils and vinegars can retain the flavors and some medicinal properties of herbs for several months to a year.

- Herbal Salts and Sugars: Create flavored salts or sugars by combining dried herbs with salt or sugar. This can retain their flavors for several months to a year. Simply mix the ingredients together and store them in airtight containers. These infused salts and sugars can add a burst of flavor to your culinary creations.

- Herbal Extracts and Tinctures: Properly prepared herbal extracts and tinctures can maintain their medicinal properties for an extended period, often several years. The duration can vary depending on the herbs used and the extraction method. Follow the guidelines in the second half of this book to prepare your herbal medicine to ensure its effectiveness and shelf life.

Remember to label and date all stored herbs and products for easy identification.

When herbs have lost their aroma and are no longer useful for culinary or medicinal purposes, there are several options for their disposal. One option is to compost them.

4   Grow your own Medicine

4.1 Introduction to Herb Gardening

Before delving into specific tips for successful plant growth in Chapter 5, let's establish the foundations of planning and maintaining your herb garden. If you already have an herb garden or indoor plants, this chapter may introduce you to some more concepts you may want to explore. However, don't overthink it! The key is to take action and gain firsthand experience in discovering what works best for you in your unique environment and what doesn't. Generally, it is more encouraging to start small and expand your herb garden (and experience) with time.

Herb Selection

The climate in the Midwest can be variable, with hot summers and cold winters. It's important to select herb varieties that are well-suited to these temperature extremes and can thrive in the region's specific growing conditions such as the ones presented in Chapter 5. Of course, indoor gardening widens the range of plants that you can grow at home and I selected the ones matching the herbal remedy-making I propose in the last part of this book.

Understanding the average frost dates and the specific requirements of different herb plants will help you plan your planting and harvesting schedules accordingly. The average frost dates in the Midwest can vary depending on the specific location within the region. However, as a general guideline, the last spring frost typically occurs between late April and early May, while the first fall frost usually happens between late September and early October.

Extreme weather conditions can pose challenges to outdoor herb gardening. Be prepared to protect your herbs from frost, heatwaves, strong winds, or heavy rain. Implement protective measures such as row covers, shade cloths, windbreaks, or mulching to safeguard your herbs from adverse conditions and maintain their health and productivity.

The Right Soil for Planting

The soil composition in the Midwest varies across the different areas. For example, areas closer to the Great Lakes may have sandy or loamy soil due to the influence of glacial deposits. On the other hand, regions further away from the lakes might have clay or silt-based soil.

Conducting a soil analysis is essential to understand the specific characteristics of your soil. The soil characteristic will determine what plants will do well in your garden or how you have to adapt the soil according to the plant's needs.

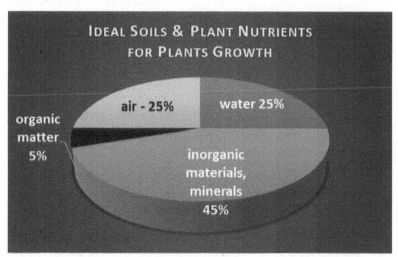

The composition of the ideal soil for plants to grow.

Source: *https://content.ces.ncsu.edu/extension-gardener-handbook/1-soils-and-plant-nutrients#section_heading_7235*

The ideal soil composition for plant growth is composed of about 50% air and water, and the other 50% is made up of inorganic materials, minerals, and organic material and microorganisms (see picture above).

I. Inorganic materials, such as sand, clay, and rock, play a crucial role in providing structure and support for plant roots. The arrangement and size of these elements determine how well the soil drains, retains water, and allows for air circulation.

II. Minerals are essential nutrients for plant growth, with 17 elements required overall. Nitrogen, phosphorus, and potassium are the primary nutrients, but other elements like calcium, iron, and magnesium are equally important. Different plants have varying needs, so it's essential to understand their specific requirements.

III. Organic matter is a vital component of living soil. Earthworms, nematodes, bacteria, and fungi work symbiotically with plants, enhancing soil structure and fertility. Decomposed plant matter and roots contribute to the overall health of the soil.

Conducting soil tests or researching the plants you are growing can help you determine what nutrients your soil lacks or has in abundance.

How to Test the Soil

Inorganic Materials: Determining the soil texture (whether it's sandy, silty, loamy, or rocky) requires a simple test that you can do by hand. Here's how to examine your soil's texture:

1. Collect soil samples: Take soil samples from different areas of your garden or planting area. Use a clean trowel or shovel to collect soil from various depths (6-8 inches deep is common).

2. Remove debris: Remove any rocks, sticks, or large clumps from the soil sample.

3. Wet the soil: Add a small amount of water to the soil sample to make it slightly moist but not waterlogged.

4. Test for texture:

o   Sandy soil: Take a handful of the moist soil and try to form a ball. Sandy soil will not hold together and will feel gritty when rubbed between your fingers.

o   Silty soil: Silty soil will form a loose ball when wet and will feel smooth when rubbed between your fingers.

o   Loamy soil: Loamy soil has the ideal texture, forming a ball that holds together but can be easily crumbled when touched.

o   Clay soil: Clayey soil will form a hard ball when wet and won't crumble easily.

5.   Observe and compare: After determining the soil texture, you can observe the overall characteristics of your soil. Sandy soil drains quickly but may require more frequent watering and fertilization. Loamy soil is well-balanced, holding nutrients and moisture while providing good drainage. Silty soil retains moisture but may need better drainage to prevent waterlogging. Clayey soil retains nutrients well but can be compacted easily.

By performing this simple test, you can get an idea of your soil's texture and make informed decisions about how to improve its structure and fertility. Remember that soil improvement can be an ongoing process, and understanding your soil's texture is the first step toward creating a healthy and productive garden.

There are several methods to determine the mineral content or essential nutrients of the soil in your garden:

•   Soil Testing Kits: Soil testing kits are available at garden centers and online. They typically come with instructions on how to collect a soil sample and perform tests for various nutrients like nitrogen, phosphorus, potassium and others as well as aicidity/alkalinity (pH). These kits are relatively simple to use and provide a basic idea of the soil's nutrient levels.

•   Soil Testing Laboratories: For more accurate and comprehensive results, you can send soil samples to a professional soil testing laboratory. Many agricultural extension offices offer soil testing services, and there are private labs as well. They will analyze your soil sample and provide detailed information on nutrient levels and recommendations for soil amendments.

- DIY Soil Testing: You can perform some simple DIY tests to get an idea of the soil's pH and nutrient content. For example, you can use a pH testing kit to determine the soil's acidity or alkalinity.

- Plant Nutrient Deficiency Symptoms: Observing your plants for nutrient deficiency symptoms can also provide some insight into the soil's nutrient status. For example, yellowing leaves may indicate a lack of nitrogen, while purple leaves may suggest phosphorus deficiency.

Remember that soil testing is essential for understanding your garden's nutrient needs accurately. By knowing the soil's nutrient profile, you can make informed decisions about fertilization and soil amendments, leading to healthier and more productive plants.

For instance, if your soil analysis reveals that your soil is sandy, you may need to amend it with organic matter such as compost or well-rotted manure to improve its moisture retention and nutrient-holding capacity.

In areas with clay soil, you might need to incorporate organic matter to enhance its drainage and prevent waterlogging. Adding materials like peat moss or perlite can help improve the soil's structure and aeration.

Determining the organic matter content of the soil in your garden can also be done through various methods:

- Visual Inspection: By observing the soil, you can get a rough estimate of its organic matter content. Dark, rich, and crumbly soil usually indicates higher organic matter content, while light-colored, sandy soil may have less organic matter.

- Feel and Texture: High organic matter soil tends to have a spongy and crumbly texture. When you squeeze it, it should hold its shape but easily break apart. Sandy soil lacks this spongy texture and tends to feel gritty.

- DIY Soil Test: You can conduct a basic DIY soil test called the "jar test." Collect a soil sample and mix it with water in a clear jar. Let the jar sit undisturbed for a few hours or overnight. Organic matter will float to the top as a dark layer or debris.

- Soil Testing Lab: For a more precise measurement of organic matter, you can send soil samples to a soil testing laboratory. They use specialized techniques to quantify the organic matter content accurately.

It is essential to know the organic matter content of your soil as it directly influences soil fertility, water-holding capacity, and overall soil health. Soils rich in organic matter support better plant growth, nutrient retention, and microbial activity. Regularly monitoring and maintaining organic matter levels in your garden soil can improve its productivity and long-term sustainability.

Garden Herb Maintenance

Garden herb maintenance encompasses several elements to ensure the health and vitality of your herbs.

Watering: Providing adequate water is crucial for herb plants. They generally prefer moist but well-drained soil. Water your herbs regularly, especially during dry periods but avoid overwatering, which can lead to root rot. When you water, aim to provide deep and thorough watering to encourage the roots to grow deeply into the soil. Water until the soil is evenly moist, but not waterlogged. Avoid shallow and frequent watering, as it can promote shallow root growth and make the plant more susceptible to drying out.

Mulching: Applying organic mulch around your herb plants helps conserve moisture, suppress weed growth, and regulate soil temperature. Mulch also adds nutrients to the soil as it breaks down.

Winter Care: In colder regions, proper winter care is essential to protect herb plants from frost or freezing temperatures. Consider covering them with mulch, burlap, or bringing potted herbs indoors to a protected area.

Consider the seasonal indications about plants:

- **Annual herbs** usually grow for just one season, from seed to plant to flower to seed.
- **Biennial herbs** complete their life cycle in 2 years, growing foliage in year 1 and going to flower and seed in year 2.
- **Perennial herbs** are those which grow for years under the right conditions. These often grow into shrubs and bushes on a balcony or in your garden. Often, they die back completely in winter but pop up again the following spring.
- **Frost hardy** means a plant will survive a cold winter outdoors.

4.2   Managing the PH of your Soils

Acidic soils have a low pH. When dealing with acidic soil, there are several effective ways to raise the pH level:

- Add Agricultural Lime: To increase pH, consider adding agricultural lime (calcium carbonate) to the soil. Follow recommendations from your soil test or gardening center for the appropriate amount to use.
- Crushed egg shells can be used for the same matter as agricultural lime and neutralize acidic soils
- Incorporate Organic Matter: Boost the soil's pH and stability by incorporating organic matter like mature compost or well-rotted manure.
- Use Wood Ash Sparingly: Wood ash from hardwood fires can also help raise pH, but use it sparingly to avoid nutrient imbalances.

Simplified PH Levels Overview

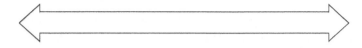

1	2	3	4	5	6	7	8	9	10	11	12	13	14
ACIDIC SOIL **pH=0: battery acid** Soils that have developed in acidic environments, such as peatlands or pine forests, will often yield pH readings below 6, indicating their acidic nature.					**SOIL PH=7 NEUTRAL** pure water			**BASIC/ ALKALINE** **pH=13: bleach** Soils that have formed in chalk or limestone environments will typically have a pH reading of 7.5 to 8, indicating their alkaline nature.					

On the other hand, if the soil is too alkaline consider following methods:

- Coffee Grounds: Coffee grounds are acidic and can help lower the pH of the soil over time. Sprinkle used coffee grounds around acid-loving plants or work them into the soil.

- Peat Moss: Peat moss is acidic and can be mixed into the soil to gradually lower pH levels.

- Pine Needles: Pine needles are acidic and can be used as a mulch around acid-loving plants to help maintain lower pH levels.

- Sulfur-Containing Amendments: Organic materials containing sulfur, such as elemental sulfur, gypsum, or sulfur-coated urea, can be added to the soil to lower pH naturally.

- Compost with Green Matter: Composting green matter like grass clippings and kitchen scraps can create a slightly acidic compost that can be added to the soil.

- Acidic Plant-based Extracts: Some natural plant extracts, like those from citrus peels, can be used to acidify the soil when applied as a liquid solution. Simply collect citrus peels from fruits like lemons or oranges. Chop or grind the peels and soak them in water for several days. Strain the liquid and dilute it with water before applying it to the soil to lower its pH and make it more acidic.

Always monitor the pH levels and adjust gradually to avoid drastic changes that could harm plants. Additionally, consider using mulch and cover crops to protect the soil and maintain a healthy pH balance over time.

4.3   Fertilizers

Herbs benefit from periodic fertilization to support their growth and productivity. In chapter 5, there are specific tips for plants that benefit from fertilization.

When fertilizing please consider:

- Choose organic fertilizers: Opt for fertilizers that are derived from natural sources, such as compost, well-rotted manure, bone meal, fish emulsion, or seaweed extract. These organic options release nutrients slowly and provide a balanced range of essential elements. For indoor gardening make sure the manure is mature to avoid pests imported into your home. Outdoors this is less important because pests like flies or worms are not harmful to the plant in an outdoor environment.

- Follow package instructions: Read and follow the instructions provided on the packaging of your chosen organic or slow-release fertilizer. The instructions will guide you on the appropriate application rates and frequency for your specific fertilizer.

- Apply fertilizers during planting (optional): Before planting your herbs, mix a small amount of organic or slow-release fertilizer into the potting mix or soil. This will provide a baseline level of nutrients for your plants as they establish their root systems.

- Supplement with top dressing: this means applying a layer of fertilizer or compost on the surface of the soil around the base of your plants while avoiding direct contact with the leaves. This layer is then gently worked into the top layer of soil or left to gradually break down and release nutrients into the soil.

- Water thoroughly after fertilizing: After applying organic fertilizers, water your container plants thoroughly to ensure the nutrients are evenly distributed and absorbed by the roots. Adequate watering helps prevent nutrient imbalances and potential root burn.

4.4 Pest Control

Pest management is vital in container gardening. Regularly inspect your plants and employ organic pest control methods whenever possible. Prevention is key to avoid infestations. Consider the following techniques:

- Handpicking: Regularly inspect your plants and manually remove any pests you find, such as aphids, caterpillars, or beetles. Wear gloves if necessary, and drop the pests into a bucket of soapy water to eliminate them.

- Neem oil: Neem oil is a natural insecticide and fungicide derived from the neem tree. Dilute neem oil according to the instructions and spray it on your plants to control pests like aphids, whiteflies, and spider mites. It disrupts their feeding and reproductive cycles.

- Insecticidal soaps: Use insecticidal soaps, which are made from natural ingredients like potassium salts of fatty acids, to control soft-bodied insects such as aphids, mealybugs, and spider mites. Follow the product instructions and spray the affected plants thoroughly.

- Homemade remedies: Create homemade pest control solutions using ingredients like garlic, onion, hot pepper, or soap. These can be mixed with water and sprayed on plants as a deterrent against pests. However, ensure you test the solution on a small portion of the plant before applying it more widely to avoid any adverse effects.

- Physical barriers: Use physical barriers like netting or floating row covers to protect your plants from pests like birds, rabbits, or insects. These barriers can be placed over the plants or around the containers to prevent direct access.

4.5 Pruning and Harvesting Techniques for Continuous Supply

Indoors as outdoors regular pruning helps maintain the shape, size, and overall health of your herb plants.

Pruning herbs involves selectively removing certain parts of the plant, such as stems, leaves, or flowers, to promote healthy growth and shape the plant. The techniques for pruning herbs can vary, but some common approaches include:

- Pinching: This involves using your fingers or pruning shears to pinch off the tips of young shoots or stems. Pinching encourages bushier growth and prevents the herb from becoming leggy.
- Cutting back: This technique involves cutting back the entire plant or specific stems to a certain height or node. It helps rejuvenate the herb, remove dead or damaged parts, and promote new growth.

Harvesting herbs involves gathering the mature parts of the plant for culinary, medicinal, or other purposes. The harvesting technique depends on the part of the herb you want to harvest. Here are some examples:

- Leaf harvesting: For herbs with edible leaves like basil or mint, you can harvest individual leaves by carefully plucking them from the stem. You can also prune entire stems with leaves attached.

- Flower harvesting: Some herbs, such as chamomile or lavender, are valued for their flowers. To harvest flowers, you can snip off the flower heads when they are fully open and at their peak.

- Seed harvesting: If you want to collect seeds, allow the plant to flower and go to seed. Once the seed heads have turned brown and dry, you can carefully cut or shake them to collect the seeds.

It's important to research the specific pruning and harvesting techniques for each herb you're growing to ensure you're doing it correctly and at the right time to maximize the plant's health and productivity.

4.6   Container Gardening

Container gardening offers several advantages, allowing herb enthusiasts to customize their growing conditions and overcome space limitations. Whether you have a small balcony, patio, or windowsill, containers provide a solution for growing herbs in various settings. You can easily create the ideal environment for specific herb varieties by controlling factors like soil composition, moisture levels, and sunlight exposure.

Selecting suitable containers and soil is crucial for successful container gardening. Consider the size, material, and drainage capabilities of containers based on the herbs you want to grow. Adequate root space, insulation, and aesthetic appeal should be taken into account. Use a high-quality potting mix or create a well-draining soil mixture to support the healthy growth of your herbs.

Adequate sunlight exposure, watering and fertilization are as important as with outdoor plants. To ensure thriving container herb gardens, you need to follow essential tips and techniques that are provided in the chapter presenting the different plants (Chapter 5).

LIKING THIS BOOK SO FAR?
GIVE US A RATING ON AMAZON!

Positive reviews from awesome customers like you help others to feel confident about choosing my book.

Could you take

60 seconds and share your happy experiences?

We will be forever grateful.

We do all we can to ensure each book is top notch. Please let us know if there are any problems or concerns to:

www.leafinprint.com
and check:
https://www.facebook.com/leafinprints
https://www.instagram.com/leafinprints/

5   Planting Herbs in the Midwest

#1   Arnica – *Arnica montana*

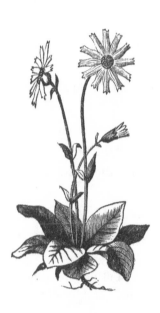

Part Used: flower heads

Taste: don't ingest!

Actions: anti-inflammatory, vulnerary

Preparation and Dosage: Topical dosage of a liniment, cream or gel, or a compress from the flowers every 4 hours for chronic pain (e.g., osteoarthritis) and every two to three hours for acute pain (e.g. Following, after surgery)

Common uses: This is a superior herb used topically for bruises and sprains. Those familiar with Arnica carry a vial of the homeopathic remedy if they fall or get a bruise. Follow the directions. As long as the skin is not broken, you can use Arnica topically for muscular rheumatic pain, arthritis, or inflammation.

Contraindications: THIS HERB IS POISONOUS. DO NOT INGEST IT UNLESS YOU TAKE IT AS A CERTIFIED HOMOEOPATHIC REMEDY FROM A CERTIFIED PRACTITIONER

Appearance: Grows to a height of 1 to 2 feet, displaying beautiful yellow, daisy-like flowers in July and August measuring 2 to 3 inches in diameter. The stems are hairy and cylindrical, ending in 1 to 3 flower stalks. The bright green leaves are slightly hairy, with toothed edges on the upper leaves and rounded tips on the lower leaves.

Native Habitat: It is native to several regions in Europe, including the mountainous areas of central and northern Europe. The plant is also found in parts of North America, such as the northern United States and Canada.

Planting Arnica:

- **Planting:** Commonly purchase established plants rather than grow them from seeds. Arnica plants can be a bit challenging to start from seeds, as they have specific germination requirements and can be slow to establish.

- **Soil:** The plant tolerates nearly any well-drained soil, but generally prefers sandy loams, slightly alkaline soil.

- **Light:** It has a preference for sunny areas but should grow fine in partially shaded areas.

- **Watering:** Arnica plants prefer moist but well-draining soil. Water the plants when the top inch of soil feels dry to the touch.

- **Fertilizing:** Not necessary for arnica, as it can thrive in nutrient-poor soils.

- **Seasonal adaptability:** Arnica is a perennial herb. It typically grows and blooms for multiple years, regenerating from the same root system each year.

- **Pruning:** Trim the aerial parts of the arnica plant, removing any dead or damaged foliage. This helps promote healthy growth.

- **Harvesting:** Arnica flowers are typically harvested when they are in full bloom. It's best to harvest them in the morning when the dew has dried but before the heat of the day. Choose flowers that are fully open and vibrant in color. After harvesting, gather the arnica flowers into small bundles and tie them securely with twine or rubber bands. Hang the bundles upside down in a well-ventilated area away from direct sunlight. This allows the flowers to dry naturally. Leave the flowers to dry for several weeks until they are fully dried. The flowers should feel crispy and brittle to the touch.

Container Gardening

If you are growing arnica in containers, you have the option to bring them indoors during winter. Place them in a cool and well-lit location, such as a greenhouse or a sunny windowsill.

#2   Basil – *Ocimum basilicum* (Sweet basil)

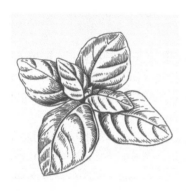

Parts Used: Leaves, flowers, and seeds

Taste: Strong, aromatic, slightly sweet

Actions: anti-inflammatory, carminative, expectorant, febrifuge

Preparation and Dosage: Culinary herb that adds vitamins and nutrients (Vitamin A, Vitamin C, calcium, phosphorus, beta carotene) to your diet for example in sauces, salads, and soups. If not prepared with food, add a couple of leaves or one tablespoon of dried basil in 2 cups of boiling water in a huge pot. Cautiously lean over the pot, cover your head with a towel and breathe in the steam for 10-15 minutes. You can also drink it as tea to reduce stress and facilitate relaxation.

Common uses: This herb has a long list of healing properties. As it is a culinary herb it is easy to consume. Consumed as tea It promotes digestion, relieves gas and bloating, aids in stress reduction, depression, acts as an antioxidant and helps the body get rid of free radicals. It reduces fever, the common cold and purifies the blood. The steam will help you with congestion and headache and will generally calm you and help with a good sleep.

Contraindications: Avoid excessive consumption during pregnancy and breastfeeding. Consult a healthcare professional before using excessively if you have any underlying medical conditions or are taking medications. The basil presented here is not Holy Basil/Tulsi (Ocimum Tenuiflorum) which has a different origin and medicinal actions. It is more difficult to grow in the Midwest than Ocimum basilicum.

Appearance: Basil plants have bright green leaves that are oval-shaped and slightly serrated. They grow as bushy plants, reaching a height of 1-2 feet, with clusters of small white or purple flowers.

Native Habitat: Basil is native to regions of Asia (India, Afghanistan, and Pakistan).

Planting Basil:

Basil, with its vibrant aroma and versatile culinary uses, is a beloved herb that thrives when grown outdoors. Its lush green leaves and aromatic profile make it a delightful addition to any garden, offering a burst of fresh flavor to countless dishes and beverages.

- **Planting:** Basil is commonly purchased as established plants rather than grown from seeds due to their specific germination requirements and slow establishment. However, the transition from the plant into home gardens can be challenging. To ensure a successful transition, it is important to acclimate the herbs gradually to their new environment. Begin by placing them in a sheltered location with indirect sunlight for a few hours each day, gradually increasing their exposure over the course of a week. After planting, closely monitor the herbs for any signs of stress or transplant shock. While it may take some time for the herbs to fully recover, following the guidelines below will help promote their successful establishment.

- **Soil:** Amend the soil with organic matter if needed, ensuring it is well-draining and nutrient-rich.

- **Light:** Basil thrives in sunny areas but can also grow in partially shaded locations.

- **Watering:** Basil prefers moist but well-draining soil. Water when the top inch of soil feels dry to the touch, providing deep watering to encourage deep root growth.

- **Fertilizing:** Basil is a moderately heavy feeder and benefits from regular fertilization. Outdoor basil plants benefit from organic mulching to help retain moisture and provide additional nutrients to the soil. If preferred, basil can be fertilized with ground coffee residue. Coffee grounds are rich in nitrogen, which is beneficial for plant growth. However, it's important to use coffee grounds in moderation and in combination with other organic fertilizers to avoid over-fertilization. Mix the coffee grounds with ordinary garden soil or compost before applying them to the soil around the basil plants. This will help improve soil fertility and provide a slow-release source of nutrients for the plants.

- **Seasonal Adaptability:** Basil is an annual herb, meaning it completes its life cycle in one growing season.

- **Pruning:** Regular pruning of basil plants promotes bushier growth and prevents flowering, which can reduce leaf production.

- **Harvesting:** Basil leaves can be harvested once the plant has reached a substantial size, typically before it begins to flower. Harvest by pinching off individual leaves or cutting stems above a leaf node.

Container Gardening:

Basil is generally grown as an annual herb, completing its lifecycle in one year. Container gardening for basil provides the advantage of year-round cultivation, allowing the herb to behave more like a perennial in a controlled indoor environment.

Planting basil in containers versus outdoor gardens has a few main differences:

- **Space:** In containers, basil plants have limited space for root growth compared to outdoor gardens. This can affect the overall size and productivity of the plant.

- **Soil:** Container gardening requires the use of potting soil, which provides good drainage and aeration for the basil plant. Outdoor gardens may have different soil types that may need amendments to ensure optimal growing conditions.

- **Watering:** Basil in containers requires more frequent watering as the soil in containers tends to dry out faster than in-ground gardens. Outdoor basil may rely more on natural rainfall.

- **Maintenance:** Container-grown basil may require more attention to pruning and fertilizing since nutrients in containers can deplete faster.

#3 Blackberry – *Rubus fruticosus*

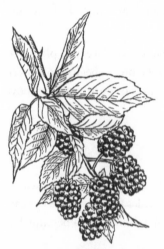

Parts Used: Berries, leaves, roots, and bark.

Taste: Berries are sweet, leaves and bark are astringent and cooling.

Actions: anti-lithic, astringent, berries are tonic

Preparation and Dosage: Standard tea dosage applies. Take one teaspoon of the dried leaves or root in boiling water. Infuse the leaves, decoct the roots. Take one cup of either leaf or root tea three times daily.

Common uses: Blackberries are good for anemia and also blood sugar stabilization. It is important to remember that most berries strengthen kidney and adrenal function.

Contraindications: Please follow the recommended dosage.

Appearance: Perennial plant that can reach a height of 3 to 6 feet. It produces clusters of small, white to pale pink flowers in late spring or early summer, which give way to delicious, dark purple or black berries. The berries are typically around 0.5 to 1 inch in length and have a sweet and tangy flavor. The plant features thorny stems that can form dense, tangled thickets, and its leaves are deep green, composed of multiple serrated leaflets.

Native Habitat: Blackberries are grown in many parts of the world, but it grows best cultivated in areas with mild winters and dry summers.

Planting Blackberry:

Blackberries are highly valued for their delicious berries and can be grown successfully in home gardens with proper care and cultivation. Blackberries are versatile and can be trained to grow on trellises or supported with stakes.

- **Soil:** Blackberries tolerate nearly any well-drained soil, but generally prefer sandy loams and slightly alkaline soil.

- **Light:** They prefer sunny areas but should grow fine in partially shaded areas.

- **Watering:** Blackberry plants prefer moist but well-draining soil.

- **Fertilizing:** Fertilize three to four weeks after planting when the plant starts growing. Fertilize at least once a year. Apply nitrogen-containing fertilizer for good growth and fruit production.

- **Seasonal adaptability:** Blackberries are perennial plants, regenerating from the same root system each year.

- **Pruning:** Trim the blackberry plant, removing any dead or damaged foliage to promote healthy growth.

- **Harvesting:** Blackberries are harvested when they are fully ripe and easily detach from the plant with a gentle tug. Pick the berries in the morning when they are cool, and the dew has dried. Handle them gently to avoid bruising and refrigerate or use them promptly after harvesting.

Container Gardening:

Blackberry can also be grown in containers. While it is typically grown as a sprawling shrub in the ground, there are compact and thornless varieties available that are suitable for container gardening. Some popular blackberry varieties for container cultivation include:

- 'Thornless Evergreen': This variety is a thornless form of *Rubus fruticosus*, making it easier to manage and harvest. It produces juicy and flavorful berries and can be grown in containers with proper support.

- 'Triple Crown': Known for its large and sweet berries, 'Triple Crown' is a thornless blackberry variety that can be successfully grown in containers. It has an upright growth habit and is suitable for smaller spaces.

- 'Navaho': This thornless variety is well-suited for container gardening due to its compact growth habit. It produces abundant crops of delicious blackberries and can be trained on a trellis or support in a container.

- 'Chester': 'Chester' is a thornless blackberry variety that is known for its late-season fruiting. It can be grown in containers and produces large, flavorful berries. It requires full sun and well-draining soil to thrive.

These varieties offer options for growing blackberries in containers, allowing individuals with limited space or who prefer container gardening to enjoy the benefits of growing their own blackberries.

#4 Black Cohosh – *Actaea racemosa*

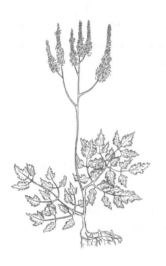

Parts Used: Root

Taste: sweet, pungent, slightly bitter, cool

Actions: antispasmodic, oxytocic

Preparation and Dosage: Standard tea dosage applies. Take one teaspoon of the dried root in one cup of boiling water three times daily.

Common uses: Black cohosh works for most nervous conditions. It relieves nerve pains and neuralgia in general. Also, it subdues the pains of childbirth and stimulates menstrual flow when it has stalled. Interestingly, it soothes coughs.

Contraindications: Please follow the recommended dosage.

Appearance: Black Cohosh is a tall perennial herb that grows 4-8 feet in height. It has dark green compound leaves with toothed leaflets, resembling a fern. The plant produces long white or cream-colored flower spikes up to 2-3 feet long blooming in late spring to early summer. The flowers are densely arranged along the spike, followed by seed pods containing black seeds.

Native Habitat: It is primarily found in deciduous forests in the eastern regions of North America and Canada. Its native range extends from the central and eastern parts of the United States, including states such as Ohio, Pennsylvania, and Maryland, to the southeastern provinces of Canada, such as Ontario and Quebec. Black Cohosh thrives in the shady understory of rich, moist woodlands and along the edges of streams and ravines.

Planting Black Cohosh:

Black Cohosh is commonly planted in gardens and cultivated for both its ornamental value and medicinal properties. It adds elegance to garden landscapes with its graceful appearance. Its attractive feathery foliage and tall, spiky flower stalks make it a popular choice for adding visual interest to shade gardens or woodland landscapes.

- Soil: Black Cohosh prefers moist, rich, and well-draining soil. It thrives in loamy or sandy soil with a slightly acidic to neutral pH level.

- Light: Partial shade to full shade is ideal for Black Cohosh. It is well-suited for growing in woodland gardens or shady areas of the garden.

- Watering: Keep the soil consistently moist but not waterlogged. Water deeply and regularly, especially during dry periods. Avoid allowing the soil to dry out completely.

- Fertilizing: Prior to the spring season, incorporating garden compost or well-aged farm manure into the soil adds necessary nutrients for the plant's well-being.

- Seasonal adaptability: Perennial herb with notable seasonal adaptability. It thrives during the spring and summer months, displaying beautiful white flower spikes. In the fall, the foliage turns a vibrant yellow before the plant enters its dormant period in winter. This resilient herb resurfaces in the following spring, showcasing its ability to adapt to changing seasons.

- Pruning: Pruning Black Cohosh is not necessary unless there are dead or damaged parts. Remove any spent flower spikes after they have finished blooming.

- Harvesting: Harvest the roots in late summer or early fall when the plant has completed its flowering stage. Carefully dig around the base of the plant and gently lift the roots from the soil. Clean the roots, remove any excess soil, and dry them thoroughly before storing.

Container Gardening:

Black Cohosh is not commonly recommended for container gardening. It is a large perennial plant that prefers to grow in the ground where it can establish a strong root system and have ample space to spread.

#5   Boneset – *Eupatorium perfoliatum*

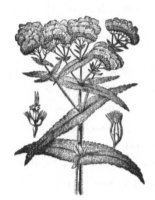

Parts Used: dried aerial parts.

Taste: very bitter

Actions: alterative, astringent, carminative, diaphoretic, expectorant, febrifuge, (laxative), tonic, vulnerary

Preparation and Dosage: Using a tincture is recommended because the tea made with this herb is too bitter. It is best to make or purchase the tincture. Tincture dosage is 1" or one dropper full three times a day for chronic conditions. In the case of acute flu symptoms or bronchial distress, you will need to take this more frequently. Take 1" every three to four hours for three days and then gradually reduce as symptoms subside. In acute cases, continue taking the chronic dosage one week after symptoms are gone.

You can make an infusion with one teaspoon of dried root per cup of boiling water. However, the tea is so bitter it may be hard to consume.

Common uses: Boneset is one of the best remedies for relieving the symptoms of influenza. This herb's pain reduction and expectorant qualities make it a superior herb — it releases chest tightness so bronchioles can drain more quickly. Additionally, it will ease constipation and provide general detoxification.

Boneset has traditionally been used to alleviate aching bones and muscles. Its name "Boneset" even originates from its historical use to help treat breakbone fever (dengue fever), a viral illness that causes severe body and bone pain.

Historically, boneset has been used as an emetic to induce vomiting for therapeutic purposes, particularly for relieving certain conditions, including constipation, stomach issues, and fever.

Contraindications: Please pay close attention to the botanical characteristics of this plant when harvesting so that you do not confuse it with Snakeroot. Boneset is safe, but Snakeroot is poisonous. The main visual difference is that the Boneset stem is hairy. Look at pictures of these two herbs carefully before you proceed.

Appearance: Boneset is a striking perennial herb with an eye-catching appearance. It features tall, upright stems that can reach heights of 3 to 5 feet. The stems are sturdy and square-shaped, with pairs of opposite leaves that appear to be joined at the base, giving it the name "perfoliatum." The leaves are lance-shaped, toothed, and have a rough texture. Atop the stems, clusters of small, white flowers bloom in late summer to early fall, forming dense, dome-shaped clusters known as corymbs.

Native Habitat: Boneset is well-adapted to the native habitats of the eastern and central United States.

Planting Boneset:

Boneset is commonly planted in gardens for its ornamental value and medicinal properties. Its attractive clusters of white flowers and foliage make it a desirable addition to flower beds, wildflower gardens, and naturalistic landscapes.

- **Soil:** Boneset thrives in moist to wet soils, particularly those with rich organic content. It prefers slightly acidic to neutral soil pH levels.

- **Light:** Boneset prefers full sun to partial shade. If grown in shaded areas, it may not flower as plentifully.

- **Watering:** Boneset requires consistently moist soil, especially during periods of active growth. It benefits from regular watering, particularly in dry spells or hot weather.

- **Fertilizing:** not required

- **Seasonal adaptability:** Boneset is a perennial herb that adapts well to seasonal changes. It grows in late spring and summer, producing small white flowers. In fall, it goes dormant, and during winter, it remains inactive. It reemerges in spring, showcasing its resilience.

- **Pruning:** Pruning is generally not necessary for Boneset. However, if the plant becomes unruly or to promote bushier growth, you can trim back the stems in early spring before new growth emerges.

- **Harvesting:** For optimal potency, harvest the plant when it is in full bloom. Handle the plant with care and use sharp scissors or pruning shears to cut the stems just above a leaf node. Harvesting should be done on a dry day to avoid excess moisture in the plant material. Dry the harvested parts in a well-ventilated area away from direct sunlight until they are fully dried and crispy.

Container Gardening:

Boneset is typically not grown in containers.

#6   Calendula – *Calendula officinalis*

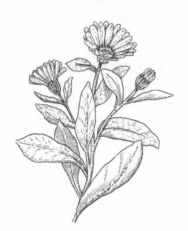

Parts Used: Flower petals, leaves

Taste: Mild, slightly bitter

Actions: Anti-inflammatory, astringent, vulnerary

Preparation and Dosage: Infuse one tablespoon of dried or two tablespoons of fresh petals on a tea ball and steep for 10-12 minutes to make an herbal tea, or use them in topical preparations such as salves, creams, or infused oils.

Common uses: Skin healing and soothing, promotes wound healing, reduces inflammation, relieves skin irritations, supports healthy menstrual cycles, and may aid in digestive discomfort.

Contraindications: Avoid internal use during pregnancy or if allergic to plants in the Asteraceae family. When planting and harvesting make sure the plants are *Calendula officinalis* and not Tagetes species, of which the French, African, and Mexican marigolds are common and have different medicinal properties.

Appearance: vibrant and cheerful annual herb known for its bright and sunny appearance. It grows up to 1 to 2 feet in height, featuring slender, green stems with pairs of opposite leaves that have a lance-like shape and a slightly hairy texture. At the tips of the stems, radiant, daisy-like flowers bloom in various shades of orange and yellow, adding a splash of color to gardens and landscapes from spring to fall.

Native Habitat: Calendula is native to the Mediterranean region but has naturalized in many temperate regions around the world.

Planting Calendula

Calendula is relatively easy to grow. It attracts pollinators and has a long blooming season, which further enhances its appeal as a garden plant.

- **Soil:** Calendula thrives in well-drained soil that is moderately fertile. It can tolerate a range of soil types, but prefers loamy or sandy soil. Ensure that the soil is not waterlogged to prevent root rot.

- **Light:** Calendula requires full sun to partial shade for optimal growth. It performs best when exposed to at least 6 hours of sunlight per day. In hotter regions, some afternoon shade may be beneficial.

- **Watering:** Calendula plants prefer regular watering to keep the soil evenly moist. Water deeply when the top inch of soil feels dry, but avoid overwatering, as it can lead to root rot. Aim for consistent moisture without waterlogging.

- **Fertilizing:** Calendula generally does not require heavy fertilization if grown in moderately fertile soil. However, a light application of a balanced organic fertilizer in early spring can provide an extra boost of nutrients.

- **Seasonal adaptability:** Calendula is an annual or short-lived perennial, depending on the climate. It is adaptable to different seasons but performs best in cool to mild temperatures.

- **Pruning:** Regular deadheading (removing spent flowers) promotes continuous blooming and prevents self-seeding. Pinching back leggy stems can also help maintain a compact and bushy habit.

- **Harvesting:** Calendula flowers are typically harvested when they are fully open and vibrant in color. Harvest them in the morning after the dew has dried but before the heat of the day. Gently pluck the flowers from the stem, and they can be used fresh or dried for various herbal preparations.

Container Gardening:

When planting Calendula (*Calendula officinalis*) in pots, choose a large container with well-draining potting soil. Place it in a sunny location and water regularly, being careful not to overwater. Fertilize every few weeks to ensure nutrient availability. Container-grown Calendula offers seasonal adaptability and can be pruned for continuous blooming.

#7   California Poppy – *Eschscholzia californica*

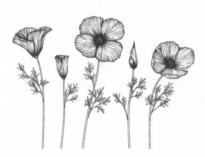

Parts Used: flowers, leaves, seeds

Taste: sweet, to slightly bitter, and astringent

Actions: anti-inflammatory, anti-spasmodic, sedative, nervine, diuretic,

Preparation and Dosage: Standard tea dosage applies. Take one teaspoon of dried flower in one cup of boiling water three times daily.

Common uses: The flower soothes anxiety, calms a nervous disposition, and induces a night of sound sleep. It could also re- move lice from hair, and reduce headaches and stomachaches. Poultices of the flower and leaves stop breast milk from flowing when the time comes for weaning a baby.

Contraindications: Please follow the recommended dosage.

Appearance: Charming flowering plant known for its vibrant and delicate appearance. The California Poppy has a compact and bushy growth habit, typically reaching a height of 12 to 18 inches. It features feathery, fern-like leaves that are bluish-green in color. The plant produces beautiful flowers that can range in color from bright yellow to orange and even deep red. Each flower has four petals and a distinct cup-shaped structure at the center. The flowers open during the day and close at night or during cloudy weather.

Native habitat: California Poppy is primarily found in California and other parts of the western United States, including Oregon, Washington, and Nevada. It is well-adapted to the dry and arid conditions of these regions, often thriving in grasslands, meadows, and open areas.

Planting California Poppy:

It is possible to cultivate California Poppy in the Midwest. It may require additional care and attention to create suitable growing conditions, as the Midwest climate and soil conditions may differ from its native habitat.

- **Soil:** California Poppy prefers well-drained soil that is sandy or loamy. It can tolerate a wide range of soil conditions, including poor or rocky soils.

- **Light:** California Poppy thrives in full sun but can tolerate partial shade. It prefers at least 6 hours of direct sunlight per day for optimal growth and flowering.

- **Watering:** California Poppy is a drought-tolerant plant and does not require excessive watering. Water the plant sparingly, allowing the soil to dry out between watering sessions. Overwatering can lead to root rot and other issues.

- **Fertilizing:** not necessary

- **Seasonal adaptability:** California Poppy is an annual or short-lived perennial plant, depending on the climate. It is well-adapted to the mild and Mediterranean climates, such as those found in California and the western United States. In colder regions, it is often grown as an annual. The plant tends to bloom from spring to early summer, producing vibrant orange, yellow, or red flowers. It may self-seed and come back the following year if growing conditions are favorable.

- **Pruning:** California Poppy does not require regular pruning. However, removing spent flowers can promote prolonged blooming and prevent self-seeding if desired. Prune any damaged or dead foliage as needed to maintain the plant's appearance.

- **Harvesting:** Harvest the leaves, stems, and flowers when they are in full bloom. Dry the harvested parts in a cool, well-ventilated area away from direct sunlight. Once fully dried, store them in airtight containers for future use in herbal preparations.

Container Gardening:

While California Poppy can be grown in containers, it is not commonly cultivated in this manner. It prefers to thrive in garden beds or natural settings, as it requires ample space for its spreading growth habit. However, if you choose to grow it in a container, select a large pot with good drainage, use a well-draining potting mix, provide ample sunlight, and water when the soil is dry. Just keep in mind that container-grown California Poppies may not reach their full potential compared to those grown directly in the ground.

#8 Chamomile – *Matricaria (chamomilla) recutita*

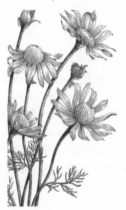

Parts Used: flowering tops

Taste: mild, floral, and slightly sweet

Actions: anti-inflammatory, carminative, expectorant, laxatives, antispasmodic, nervine, vulnerary

Preparation and dosage: Standard tea dosage applies. Take one teaspoon of the dried flower in one cup of boiling water three times daily.

Common uses: Chamomile benefits are numerous for children and adults. Chamomile alleviates insomnia, anxiety, depression, appetite, menopausal mood swings, diarrhea, aches and pains from flu, migraines, motion sickness, vertigo, conjunctivitis, skin inflammations, and a host of digestive symptoms such as gas, colic pains, or even ulcers.

Contraindications: If you are allergic to ragweed, you will probably be allergic to this plant. Compresses with Chamomile have occasionally produced a rash. In most cases, it is very gentle and safe.

Appearance: Small, daisy-like flower with a bright yellow center and delicate white petals. It typically grows to a height of 12 to 24 inches, forming a compact and bushy plant.

Native Habitat: German Chamomile is common and does well in poor, clay soil, whereas the Roman variety prefers well-drained and moderately fertile soil. Both types, however, thrive in open, sunny locations. Its cousin, *Pineapple Weed,* grows in gravel and sandy areas (such as driveways). Pineapple Weed is easier to find than true Chamomile yet has similar medicinal benefits. Pineapple weed is milder.

Planting Chamomile:

Chamomile is a versatile herb that can thrive in various growing conditions.

- **Soil:** Chamomile prefers well-drained, moderately fertile soil. It can tolerate a range of soil types but thrives in loamy or sandy soil.
- **Light:** Chamomile thrives in full sun but can also tolerate partial shade. It typically requires at least 6 hours of direct sunlight per day.
- **Watering:** Chamomile plants prefer regular watering to keep the soil evenly moist but not waterlogged.
- **Fertilizing:** not required
- **Seasonal adaptability:** Chamomile is an annual herb that adapts well to various seasons. It is typically sown in spring and harvested in summer.

- **Pruning:** Pruning chamomile is not necessary for its growth. However, removing spent flowers can encourage continuous blooming and prevent self-seeding.

- **Harvesting:** Chamomile flowers can be harvested when they are fully open and vibrant. The best time to harvest is in the morning after the dew has dried but before the heat of the day. Gather the flowers and dry them for use in teas or other herbal preparations.

Container Gardening:

Chamomile is well-suited for container gardening. Just use a well-draining potting mix.

#9   Comfrey – *Symphytum officinale*

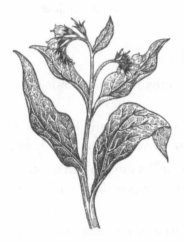

Parts Used: Leaves, roots

Taste: Do not ingest!

Actions: Anti-inflammatory, Astringent, Vulnerary

Preparation and Dosage: Comfrey can be used externally as a poultice, salve, or herbal compress for wounds, bruises, sprains, and skin conditions.

Common uses: Traditionally used for promoting wound healing, reducing inflammation, arthritis, soothing skin irritations, and supporting bone and joint health.

Contraindications: Internal use should be avoided due to potential liver toxicity and the presence of pyrrolizidine alkaloids. Avoid applying comfrey to open wounds or broken skin. Not recommended for use during pregnancy or breastfeeding. Talk to a medicinal practitioner before giving it to children or if you had a history of liver disease.

Appearance: Comfrey is a perennial herb with hairy, lance-shaped leaves that are dark green in color. It typically reaches a height of 2 to 4 feet and forms a clump of broad, lance-shaped leaves. The plant grows upright with bell-shaped flowers that can be white, pink, or purple.

Native Habitat: Comfrey is native to Europe and parts of Asia but has naturalized in many regions worldwide. It prefers moist, fertile soil and can be found in gardens, meadows, and along streams or riverbanks.

Planting Comfrey:

Comfrey is a hardy perennial herb that can thrive in various growing conditions. However, it is important to note that Comfrey can be invasive if not properly contained, so it is recommended to grow it in a designated area or use containers to control its spread.

- **Soil:** Comfrey prefers fertile, well-draining soil. It can tolerate various soil types, but it thrives in moist and nutrient-rich soil.

- **Light:** Comfrey grows best in full sun to partial shade. It can tolerate some shade, but it may affect its growth and productivity.

- **Watering:** Comfrey has moderate water needs. Keep the soil consistently moist but avoid overwatering, as it can lead to root rot. Water deeply when the top inch of soil feels dry.

- **Fertilizing:** Comfrey is a nutrient accumulator, meaning it can draw nutrients from the soil and store them in its leaves. It generally doesn't require additional fertilization, but incorporating organic matter into the soil during planting can be beneficial.

- **Seasonal adaptability:** Comfrey is a hardy perennial that can adapt to different seasons. It goes dormant during winter and regrows in spring. It is generally cold-tolerant but may need protection in harsh winter conditions.

- **Pruning:** Comfrey can grow vigorously, and regular pruning helps maintain its shape and prevent it from becoming invasive.

Cut back the plant after flowering to encourage new growth and prevent self-seeding.

- **Harvesting:** The leaves of Comfrey are typically harvested during the growing season. Harvesting can be done by cutting the mature leaves near the base of the plant. Avoid harvesting all the leaves at once, allowing the plant to continue growing and producing new foliage.

Container Gardening:

Comfrey can be grown in containers, but it's important to choose a large and deep container to accommodate its extensive root system. A container with a minimum depth of 12 inches is recommended. Make sure the container has good drainage to prevent waterlogging, as Comfrey prefers moist but well-draining soil. Container-grown Comfrey may require more frequent watering compared to those grown in the ground. Additionally, regular pruning and maintenance are necessary to control the plant's size and prevent it from becoming too large for the container.

#10 Dandelion – *Taraxacum officinale*

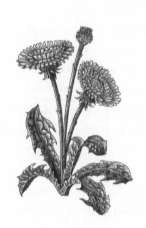

Parts Used: flowers, leaves, roots

Taste: bitter to bittersweet, astringent

Actions: alterative, tonic, diuretic, hepato-protective, depurative, carminative, hepatics

Preparation and Dosage: Standard tea dosage applies. Take one teaspoon of dried flower, leaf or root, in one cup of boiling water three times daily.

Common uses: Dandelion is one herb that can cause improvement in almost any condition. Poultices from the roots reach into an infection and reduce it. The leaves stimulate appetite and digestion. They assist with calcium absorption. Dandelion moves blood, so understandably, it benefits liver and gallbladder stagnation. It relieves premenstrual syndrome because it decongests the blood.

Contraindications: Please follow the recommended dosage. Drink plenty of water when consuming this herb to facilitate detoxification.

Appearance: Perennial herb with a distinctive appearance. It features a basal rosette of deeply toothed, lance-shaped leaves that can grow up to 12 inches long. From the center of the rosette emerges a hollow, leafless stem that can reach a height of 12 to 18 inches. At the top of the stem, bright yellow composite flowers form a round, globe-like cluster. These flowers consist of numerous small petals surrounded by green bracts. After blooming, dandelions produce fluffy, spherical seed heads known as "dandelion clocks" that disperse their seeds by wind.

Native Habitat: Dandelions thrive on neglect. It is native to Europe and Asia but its ability to colonize different ecosystems makes it a familiar sight in many parts of the world.

Planting in Gardens and Containers:

Dandelions are typically not intentionally planted in gardens or pots, as they are considered weeds by many gardeners. But the chances are high you will find them in your garden or public area.

#11 Echinacea – *Echinacea* spp.

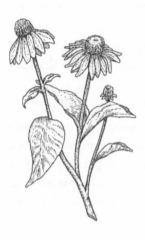

Parts Used: root and aerial portions

Actions: alterative, antibiotic, carminative, stimulant, vulnerary

Preparation and Dosage: Take the Standard Infusion 1 teaspoon of dried leaves and flowers per cup of boiling water. Drink three cups daily. This herb tinctures well and is worth keeping on hand. For chronic, long-term ailments, take 1" of tincture in the morning and evening. For acute conditions like severe inflammation or infections, you will take 1" or one dropper full every three hours until symptoms subside. Then decrease the dosage slowly as you ease into the chronic phase.

Common uses: Echinacea is widely available online due to its popularity. Echinacea alleviates even the most severe inflammatory conditions: boils, skin eruptions, puffy sores, venomous bites, gangrene septicemia, poison oak, and poison ivy. As an antibacterial or antiviral medicine, it is also superior. Within three days of taking the *acute dosage* of Echinacea, acute pus or inflammation should subside, as well as any acute bacterial or viral infections. It is an excellent lymphatic cleanser.

Contraindications: Follow the recommended dosage always. This herb is used longer-term, up to six months, very safely.

Appearance: Perennial herb that typically grows to a height of 2 to 4 feet. It features erect, sturdy stems with rough texture and can produce multiple branching stems. The leaves are dark green, lance-shaped, and have a coarse texture. Echinacea flowers are daisy-like, with vibrant petals that range in color from pink, purple, or white. The center of the flower is cone-shaped and spiky, giving it a unique appearance.

Native Habitat: Echinacea comes in 9 different species, all of which are native to North America.

Planting Echinacea:

Echinacea is a versatile plant that can be grown in gardens and pots.

- **Soil:** Echinacea prefers well-drained, loamy soil that is rich in organic matter. It can tolerate a range of soil conditions but thrives in moderately fertile soil.

- **Light:** Echinacea requires full sun to partial shade. It performs best when exposed to at least 6 hours of direct sunlight per day.

- **Watering:** Echinacea is drought-tolerant once established and prefers moderate moisture levels. Water the plant deeply but infrequently, allowing the soil to dry slightly between watering.

- **Fertilizing:** Echinacea generally does not require heavy fertilization. However, incorporating compost or well-rotted manure into the soil before planting can provide essential nutrients.

- **Seasonal adaptability:** Echinacea is a hardy perennial that is adaptable to a range of climates. It can tolerate both hot summers and cold winters.

- **Pruning:** Deadheading spent flowers can promote prolonged blooming and prevent self-seeding. Prune back the entire plant in late fall or early spring to encourage new growth.

- **Harvesting:** For flowers, harvest when they are fully open and vibrant. For roots, harvest in the fall after the plant has reached maturity. Dry the harvested parts thoroughly before storing.

Container Gardening:

Choose a deep container to accommodate the taproot of Echinacea. Container-grown Echinacea may require more frequent watering and fertilization and may require additional winter protection.

#12 Elderberry – *Sambucus nigra*

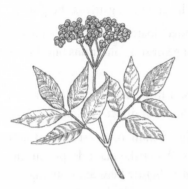

Parts Used: berries, roots, inner bark, leaves.

Taste: sweet, sour, slightly astringent

Actions: antiviral, adaptogenic, anti-inflammatory, cardiotonic, diaphoretic, alterative, emollient

Preparation and Dosage: Standard tea dosage applies. Take one teaspoon of the dried fruit in one cup of boiling water three times daily for ear, nose, and throat issues or flu. Take one teaspoon of the dried root in one cup of boiling water two times daily for constipation. Take one teaspoon of syrup found in the recipe section three times daily in a chronic case of sore throat, cough, or cold. For any critical ailment, such as the flu or bronchitis, take the syrup every three hours.

Common uses: Elderberry is a medicine chest must-have for a family. It excels in treating cough, bronchitis, flu, fever, and colds. In general, it reduces inflammation and is an excellent antiviral remedy for children and adults alike. A tea from the bark relieves constipation. The berries help arthritis. It is an ideal herb for children, mainly because they love the taste of syrup. The berries provide strength for adrenal function, as most berries do.

Contraindications: Please follow the recommended dosage.

Appearance: Tall deciduous shrub, reaching heights of 10-12 feet. It features serrated dark green leaves and produces clusters of small, creamy white flowers in spring, followed by dark purple to black berries in late summer. The bark of elderberry is grayish-brown and has a rough texture.

Native Habitat: Elderberry is common throughout plains and mountains in northern and western regions. It is found in wetlands and along streams in the east.

Planting Elderberry:

In gardens, it is often planted as a shrub or used for hedging due to its size and attractive appearance.

- **Soil:** Elderberries prefer well-draining soil that is rich in organic matter. They can tolerate a range of soil types but thrive best in loamy or sandy soil.

- **Light:** Elderberries prefer full sun for optimal growth and fruit production. They can tolerate some shade but may produce fewer flowers and fruits in shaded areas.

- **Watering:** Elderberries have moderate water needs and prefer consistently moist soil. They should be watered regularly, especially during dry periods.

- **Fertilizing:** Elderberries benefit from regular fertilization with a balanced, slow-release fertilizer in early spring. This helps promote healthy growth and fruit development.

- **Seasonal adaptability:** Elderberries are deciduous shrubs that are adapted to temperate climates. They are able to withstand cold winters.

- **Pruning:** Pruning elderberries is important for maintaining their shape, promoting air circulation, and rejuvenating the plant. Prune in late winter or early spring when the plant is dormant.

- **Harvesting:**
  o Elderberry berries: Harvest fully ripe clusters of dark purple or black berries, using clean pruners or scissors.

  o Elderberry roots: Dig up the dormant plant during late fall or early spring, preserving as much of the root system as possible.

  o Elderberry inner bark: Carefully peel away the outer bark using a sharp knife, starting at the base and working your way up.

  o Elderberry leaves: Select mature leaves in the morning, plucking them gently from the stem, and rinse before air drying.

Container Gardening:

Dwarf or compact varieties of elderberry can be selected to accommodate limited space and provide an ornamental touch to patios or balconies.

When planted in containers, elderberries require larger-sized pots or containers to accommodate their root system. The containers should have good drainage to prevent waterlogging. Container-grown elderberries may require more frequent watering as the soil in containers tends to dry out faster. Adequate sunlight is crucial, so containers should be placed in a sunny location. Fertilization may need to be adjusted since container-grown plants have limited access to nutrients in the surrounding soil. Pruning is still necessary to maintain the plant's shape and health.

#13 Wild Ginger – *Asarum canadense*

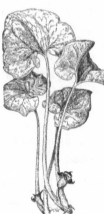

Parts Used: root

Taste: pungent

Actions: anti-inflammatory, antitussive, antiviral, carminative, cardiotonic, diaphoretic, expectorant, hypotensive, rubefacient, tonic

Preparation and Dosage: An infusion can be made from one teaspoonful of the fresh root in one cup of boiling water and taken whenever needed as a tonic herb, or at least three times a day for cold, cough, or flu.

Common uses: Ginger relieves morning sickness, chemotherapy-associated nausea, postoperative nausea, and motion sickness. Ginger can potentially treat several ailments, including degenerative disorders such as arthritis and rheumatism, indigestion, constipation and ulcer, and cardiovascular conditions like atherosclerosis and hypertension. On the whole, Ginger contains remarkable anti-inflammatory and anti-oxidative properties for controlling the process of aging.

Contraindications: Ginger is a tonic and adaptogenic herb that can be used regularly with no contraindications. However, do not take this herb if you suffer from hot flashes. It creates heat.

ATTENTION: While wild ginger (*Asarum canadense*) and ordinary ginger (*Zingiber officinale*) share the name "ginger," they are different plant species with distinct characteristics and medicinal properties. Ordinary ginger, which is commonly used in culinary and herbal applications, is known for its anti-inflammatory, digestive, and immune-boosting properties. It is often used to treat nausea, indigestion, and inflammation-related conditions.

Wild ginger, also known as Canadian ginger, has a different set of medicinal properties. It is traditionally used as a digestive aid and for its mild stimulating effects on the digestive system. Wild ginger is not typically used in the same way as ordinary ginger in culinary applications or for its anti-inflammatory properties and is toxic if consumed in very high quantities.

Appearance: Low-growing perennial herb that typically reaches a height of 6 to 10 inches. It has heart-shaped leaves that are dark green and glossy, with prominent veins. The leaves grow in pairs from the base of the plant and can form a dense groundcover. The plant produces small, brownish-purple flowers that are hidden beneath the foliage and not easily noticed. The rhizomes of wild ginger have a spicy, ginger-like aroma when crushed, giving the plant its common name. Rhizomes are rootlike, often thickened, and usually horizontal underground plant stems that produces shoots above and roots below

Native Habitat: The native habitat of wild ginger (*Asarum canadense*) includes woodland areas and shady, moist environments in eastern North America. It is native to regions such as the Midwest, Northeast, and Southeast of the United States, as well as parts of Canada.

Planting Ginger:

While it is native to the region and can be found growing naturally in woodland areas, it is less frequently grown in home gardens. This is partly due to its specific growth requirements and less widespread availability in the horticultural market. But you can still give it a try:

- **Planting:** Wild ginger is commonly planted from the rhizome as growing it from the seeds is complicated. Early spring is the best time to divide wild ginger from the forest as new growth appears. Otherwise, you may just order the rhizomes online. Then, just put the roots horizontally into a container and cover with rich soil like compost.

- **Soil:** Wild ginger thrives in rich, moist, and well-draining soil. It prefers loamy or sandy soil with ample organic matter.

- **Light:** Wild ginger is typically found in shady woodland areas. It prefers partial to full shade and can tolerate deep shade.

- **Watering:** Keep the soil consistently moist but not waterlogged. Regular watering is necessary, especially during dry periods.

- **Fertilizing:** Wild ginger generally does not require regular fertilization. However, incorporating organic matter such as leaf mulch or compost into the soil can provide nutrients.

- **Seasonal adaptability:** Wild ginger is a native perennial plant in the Midwest and is adapted to the local climate. It can withstand cold winters and can thrive in different seasons. Be cautious about snails or slugs that damage the plants especially in early spring.

- **Pruning:** Minimal pruning is needed for wild ginger. Remove any dead or damaged leaves as necessary.

- **Harvesting:** To harvest Wild ginger without killing the plant just dig up the rhizomes, snip off short pieces of the rhizome just between the plant, and re-plant the parts that have roots. By carefully selecting and trimming the desired portions, you can gather the harvested pieces for further processing or immediate use.

Container Gardening:

When cultivated in containers, consider using one with good drainage and ample space for the plant to spread. Provide well-draining, organic-rich soil, and place the pot in a shady location. Keep the soil consistently moist, fertilize as needed, and perform minimal pruning.

#14 American Ginseng – *Panax quinquefolius*

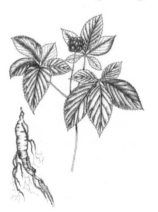

Parts Used: root

Actions: adaptogenic, tonic, stimulant

Taste: slightly bitter

Preparation and Dosage: Using the Ginseng root, make a decoction from half a teaspoon of the dried root. It is best to start small with this herb. Take ½ teaspoon in a cup of boiling water three times daily.

Common uses: It is a powerful adaptogen with a wide range of possible therapeutic uses. It has a tremendous therapeutic application for the weak, the lethargic, and the elderly. Ginseng has an ancient history. It was a sexual tonic and aided various conditions like headaches, digestive distress, and female infertility.

Contraindications: Acute inflammatory diseases and bronchitis, headaches, and insomnia. American Ginseng is overly stimulating for these conditions due to its invigorating quality.

Appearance: Perennial herb that grows to a height of about 12-24 inches. It has compound leaves with five leaflets, each leaflet being ovate in shape and pointed at the tip. The plant produces small clusters of greenish-white flowers in the summer, which are followed by bright red berries in the fall.

Native Habitat: Native to the eastern regions of North America, including the United States and Canada. It is commonly found in the deciduous forests of the Appalachian and Ozark Mountain ranges, as well as other shaded and moist woodland areas. Due to overharvesting, American Ginseng is now considered a threatened species in the wild and is protected by regulations in many areas.

Planting American Ginseng:

This plant can be cultivated in gardens by mimicking its natural habitat.

Planting: The simplest method of planting ginseng is by using the root itself. The best planting season for ginseng is typically in the fall, preferably in September or October. During this time, the soil is still warm, which allows the ginseng seeds or roots to establish and develop a strong root system before winter. Plant the root at a slight angle (30-45° from vertical) with the bud positioned approximately an inch below the soil surface. Space the plants 4-6 inches apart within rows that are 6-12 inches apart. Apply a layer of mulch several inches thick. Initially, the young shoots may be barely visible when they emerge.

Light: American Ginseng prefers shaded or partially shaded areas. It thrives under a dense canopy of trees or shade structures to protect it from direct sunlight.

Watering: American Ginseng requires consistent moisture in the soil. It should be watered regularly to keep the soil evenly moist but not waterlogged.

Fertilizing: American Ginseng benefits from organic fertilizers, such as compost or well-rotted manure, applied during the growing season. Fertilization helps provide essential nutrients for healthy growth.

Seasonal adaptability: American Ginseng is adapted to temperate regions and goes through a dormancy period during winter. It requires a cold period for germination and specific temperature conditions throughout the growing season.

Pruning: Pruning is generally not necessary for American Ginseng. However, removing any dead or diseased leaves or stems can help maintain plant health.

Harvesting: It takes several years for the roots to develop fully and reach their desired size and potency. Therefore, the roots are typically harvested after at least 5-6 years of growth. Harvesting the roots before they have matured may not yield the desired medicinal properties.

Container Gardening:

Planting American Ginseng in containers is less common compared to outdoor cultivation. When planting ginseng in containers, key differences include selecting a suitable container size, providing shade or partial shade, managing watering and moisture levels, and ensuring proper nutrient supply. Harvesting follows similar guidelines as outdoor cultivation.

#15 Goldenrod – *Solidago* spp.

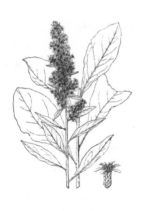

Parts Used: aerial parts

Taste: Slightly bitter, aromatic, slightly sweet

Actions: astringent, stimulating, diaphoretic, diuretic, antiseptic, anti-inflammatory, analgesic

Preparation and Dosage: Make a Standard Infusion: 1 teaspoon dried herb (aerial parts) per cup of boiling water. Drink three cups daily.

Common uses: Goldenrod uses vary from relieving influenza, calming repeated colds, soothing bronchitis, or treating tonsillitis, sinusitis, and allergies. It is mainly a respiratory herb. Ironically, many people suffer from Goldenrod allergies. However, being introduced to a tablespoon at a time of the tea over the summer months, while the plant is blooming can sometimes alleviate seasonal Fall allergies.

Contraindications: Do not take this herb if you have heart or kidney failure. It has a strong diuretic quality.

Appearance: Perennial plant that typically grows to a height of 2 to 4 feet. It features long, slender stems with clusters of small, yellow flowers. The flowers form dense, elongated plumes or spikes that give the plant a visually striking appearance. The leaves are usually lance-shaped and often have serrated edges. Goldenrod is known for its vibrant and showy display of yellow flowers, which attract pollinators like bees and butterflies.

Native Habitat: There are more than 125 species of Goldenrod, most of them native to North America for hundreds of years. You will find it in the sun to part shade, meadows and fields. Goldenrod seeds proliferate. Notice the term *Solidago* spp. meaning solid. The medicine made from it reputedly made you solid or healthy again.

Planting Goldenrod:

Its vibrant yellow flowers and tall, upright growth make it a popular choice for adding color and texture to flower beds and borders. Additionally, goldenrod is known for attracting pollinators, such as bees and butterflies, making it a beneficial addition to garden ecosystems.

Light: Goldenrod prefers full sun to partial shade for optimal growth and medicinal potency.

Watering: Goldenrod has moderate water needs and prefers well-drained soil. Water the plant when the top inch of soil feels dry.

Fertilizing: Goldenrod generally doesn't require heavy fertilization. However, adding organic matter or a balanced fertilizer during the growing season can promote healthy growth.

Seasonal Adaptability: Goldenrod is a hardy perennial plant that adapts well to different seasons. It can tolerate both hot summers and cold winters.

Pruning: Pruning goldenrod is not necessary for medicinal purposes unless you want to manage its size or shape. Remove any dead or damaged foliage to maintain plant health.

Harvesting: For medicinal use, harvest the aerial parts of goldenrod when the plant is in full bloom. Dry the harvested plant material in a well-ventilated area, away from direct sunlight, until it is crispy and can be easily crumbled. Store the dried goldenrod in an airtight container for future use in herbal preparations.

Container Gardening:

While goldenrod can be grown in containers, it is less common compared to its cultivation in garden beds or natural landscapes. Goldenrod plants can grow quite tall and have extensive root systems, which may require larger containers to accommodate their size. Additionally, goldenrod is a perennial plant that can spread quickly through rhizomes, making it more suitable for open garden spaces where it can naturalize.

#16 Horsetail – *Equisetum arvense*

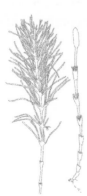

Parts Used: dried aerial stems

Taste: astringent, neutral to slightly bitter

Actions: astringent, diuretic, tonic, vulnerary

Preparation and dosage: Make a tea using one teaspoon of the dried stems per cup of boiling water. Take this three times daily. This herb does not tincture very well.

Common uses: This herb is a mild diuretic. It tones and acts as an astringent for the genitourinary system. It makes a good poultice because it contains silica, an essential mineral that strengthens all connective tissues and heals the skin. Horsetail fortifies the kidneys. It works for incontinence and bed-wetting with children.

Contraindications: Please follow the recommended dosage. There is a slight possibility of ingesting toxins if you overdose in large quantities. It is better to use this herb under the guidance of a practitioner.

Appearance: Horsetail is a perennial plant characterized by its distinctive appearance. It features hollow, segmented stems resembling bamboo or horsetail tails, reaching heights of 1 to 4 feet. The stems are covered in small, scale-like structures and lack true leaves. Horsetail produces cone-like structures called strobili for reproduction. Due to its invasive nature requires caution in planting and containment.

Native Habitat: Horsetail grows in rocky or sandy, well-drained soil, often along the road's edge in forested areas. It can also grow in more swampy conditions. It is an unmistakable herb that dates back to the Paleozoic Era. The sturdy stalks extend upwards with large needle-like projections fanning out from around the circumference of the stem. Early settlers used this plant to scrub pots and pans!

Planting Horsetail:

Horsetail has a tendency to spread quickly and can become difficult to control, which makes it less popular among gardeners. However, some gardeners may choose to grow it in contained areas or pots to prevent its spread and enjoy its unique appearance.

However, you may find it growing wild in your garden or public areas.

#17 Lavender – *Lavandula angustifolia*

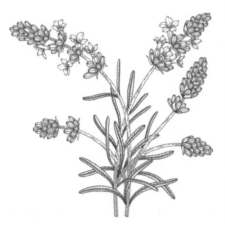

Parts Used: Flowers,

Taste: Floral, aromatic

Actions: Anti-inflammatory, sedative

Preparation and Dosage: Lavender can be used in various forms, including dried flowers, essential oil, and herbal preparations. It is commonly used in aromatherapy, infused oils, herbal teas, and topical applications such as creams and salves.

Common uses: To make lavender tea, steep 1 teaspoon of dried lavender flowers or 2 teaspoons of fresh lavender flowers in boiling water for 5-10 minutes. Strain and sweeten if desired. Enjoy warm or chilled. Lavender is renowned for its calming and relaxing properties. It is often used to promote restful sleep, reduce anxiety and stress, soothe headaches, and alleviate mild pain and inflammation. It is also valued for its aromatic qualities and is frequently used in perfumes, soaps, and beauty products.

Contraindications: Lavender is generally considered safe for most individuals when used topically or in aromatherapy. However, some individuals may experience skin irritation or allergic reactions. It is always recommended to perform a patch test before using lavender products on the skin. Internal use of lavender oil or ingestion of large quantities should be avoided. Avoid high doses during pregnancy.

Appearance: Lavender (*Lavandula angustifolia*) is a small to medium-sized perennial plant that typically grows to a height of 1 to 3 feet. It has slender, woody stems with narrow, gray-green leaves. Lavender plants can have a spread or width of about 1 to 2 feet, creating a compact and bushy appearance.

Native Habitat: Lavender is native to the Mediterranean region but is cultivated in various parts of the world.

Planting Lavender:

Lavender is commonly found in gardens, particularly in temperate climates.

- **Light:** Lavender requires full sun and at least 6-8 hours of direct sunlight per day.
- **Watering:** Lavender prefers well-drained soil and is drought-tolerant once established. Water sparingly and allow the soil to dry out between waterings.
- **Fertilizing:** Lavender generally doesn't require much fertilizer. If needed, a slow-release balanced fertilizer can be applied in spring.
- **Seasonal adaptability:** Lavender is a perennial herb that is well-adapted to various seasons, but it may require winter protection in colder regions.
- **Pruning:** Regular pruning is important to maintain the shape and health of the lavender plant. Prune in early spring or after flowering to remove spent blooms and promote bushier growth.
- **Harvesting:** Harvest lavender flowers when they are fully open and just before they start to fade. Cut the flower stems near the base and hang them upside down to dry.

Container Gardening:

The advantage of container gardening is the ability to easily adapt to seasonal changes by moving the plant as needed. Choose a larger container to allow for proper root development and use a well-draining potting mix and be mindful of more frequent watering needs. Container-grown lavender may benefit from occasional fertilization.

#18 Lemon Balm – *Melissa officinalis*

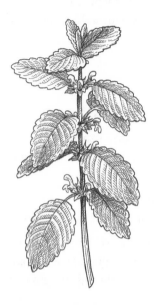

Parts Used: aerial parts

Taste: aromatic

Actions: adaptogenic, anti-inflammatory, carminative, nervine, antispasmodic, diaphoretic, antimicrobial, hepatic

Preparation and Dosage: Make a Standard Infusion with one teaspoon of the dried herb or in a cup of boiling water. Take three cups daily.

Common uses: Like Chamomile, Lemon Balm is a superior herb for digestive spasms. It helps with anxiety or depression symptoms and effects from tension or neuralgia. It relieves palpitations coming from anxiety or insomnia.

This plant interfaces between the digestive tract and nervous system. This is an action of high value because it is a neurorestorative herb and digestive tonic herb, all at once. Lemon Balm works well for headaches. It also aids the heart and circulatory system. As a vasodilator, it will lower blood pressure. When you have the flu, this herb is a great companion as it has excellent antiviral properties. It can alleviate feverish conditions while calming the nerves. Its antimicrobial components are noteworthy. Lemon Balm is one of the best herbs to keep for children.

Contraindications: Follow the recommended dosage. It is a very gentle herb. It can easily be used with the elderly and also with children.

Appearance: Perennial herb that typically grows to a height of 1 to 2 feet. It features vibrant green leaves that are heart-shaped and have a distinct lemon scent when crushed. The plant produces small clusters of white or pale yellow flowers that attract bees and other pollinators. Lemon Balm has a bushy and spreading growth habit, with stems that can become woody over time.

Native Habitat: Native to the Mediterranean region, specifically southern Europe and the Middle East. It is well adapted to warm climates and can be found growing wild in areas with mild winters and abundant sunlight.

Planting Lemon Balm:

Lemon balm is a popular plant grown in herb gardens.

- **Light:** Lemon Balm prefers full sun to partial shade. It thrives in bright light conditions, but some shade during hot summer afternoons can be beneficial.

- **Watering:** Keep the soil consistently moist but not waterlogged. Water the plant deeply whenever the top inch of soil feels dry.

- **Fertilizing:** Lemon Balm does not require heavy fertilization. Incorporate organic matter into the soil before planting and apply a balanced organic fertilizer once or twice during the growing season.

- **Seasonal adaptability:** Lemon Balm is a hardy perennial that adapts well to different seasons. It can withstand mild frosts and is typically dormant during the winter.

- **Pruning:** Regular pruning helps maintain the compact shape of the plant and promotes bushier growth. Prune Lemon Balm regularly to remove spent flowers and keep the plant tidy.

- **Harvesting:** Harvest the leaves of Lemon Balm as needed by snipping off the individual leaves or cutting back entire stems. The leaves are most flavorful before the plant flowers. For medicinal use, harvest the leaves when the essential oil content is at its highest, typically in the morning after the dew has dried.

Container Gardening:

Container gardening with Lemon Balm is popular and offers several advantages. It allows individuals with limited space or no garden access

UNLOCK THE SECRETS OF PLANT MEDICINE AT HOME

to grow this herb. When growing Lemon Balm in containers, there are a few differences to note compared to outdoor gardening. Containers should have good drainage and be large enough to accommodate the plant's root system. Ensure the container receives adequate sunlight and provide consistent watering to keep the soil moist. Fertilize the plant as needed and consider using a well-draining potting mix. Pruning and harvesting methods remain the same as outdoor gardening.

#19 Marshmallow – *Althaea officinalis*

Parts Used: root, leaves, flowers

Taste: Mild, slightly sweet

Actions: anti-inflammatory, diuretic, expectorant

Preparation and Dosage:

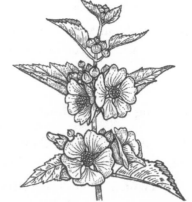

- Marshmallow root can be prepared as an herbal infusion, decoction, or as a powdered form. To make the infusion, add 1 tablespoon of Marshmallow root in 1 cup on warm, not boiling water and steep for 10 minutes. Drink a few cups of marshmallow tea throughout the day.

- The fresh, crushed flowers can be boiled for 2 minutes in hot water and then be applied warm to soothe inflamed skin to alleviate local irritation.

- You can collect a couple of leaves, add 2 cups of water and steep for 10 minutes to prepare Infusions.

Common uses: Marshmallow is often used for its soothing and moisturizing properties. It is commonly used to relieve sore throat, coughs, and respiratory discomfort. It is also valued for its demulcent properties, which help to soothe and protect the mucous membranes of the digestive and urinary systems (bladder infection, frequent urination). Marshmallow is also used topically to soothe skin irritations and promote wound healing. Gargle this infusion to soothe sore throats and gum inflammations.

Contraindications: Marshmallow is typically considered safe when used as directed, including during pregnancy. However, individuals with diabetes should be vigilant in monitoring their blood sugar levels, as Marshmallow may have an impact on glucose regulation.

Appearance: Marshmallow is a perennial herb that grows up to 4-5 feet in height. It has a thick, fleshy taproot and hairy, soft leaves that are gray-green in color. The plant produces clusters of pale pink or white flowers with five petals.

Native Habitat: Marshmallow is native to Europe, North Africa, and Western Asia. It is commonly found in wetlands, marshes, and damp meadows.

Planting Marshmallow:

The Midwest's temperate climate and suitable growing conditions provide an ideal environment for Marshmallow to thrive.

- **Light:** Marshmallow prefers full sun to partial shade. It thrives in bright, indirect light.
- **Watering:** Marshmallow requires regular watering to keep the soil consistently moist. Avoid overwatering, as it may lead to root rot.
- **Fertilizing:** Marshmallow benefits from organic fertilizers, such as compost or well-rotted manure, applied during the growing season to promote healthy growth.
- **Seasonal adaptability:** Marshmallow is a perennial plant that adapts well to the seasonal changes in the Midwest. It goes dormant during the winter and regrows in the spring.

- **Pruning:** Pruning is not typically necessary for Marshmallow, but you can remove any dead or damaged stems to maintain its overall health and appearance.

- **Harvesting:** The roots and leaves of Marshmallow are harvested for medicinal purposes. The roots are typically harvested in the fall after the plant has flowered, while the leaves can be harvested throughout the growing season. The flowers are in bloom during August and September and can then be harvested.

Container Gardening:

Container-grown Marshmallow requires a suitable-sized pot with good drainage, as opposed to being planted directly in the ground. The limited space in containers may affect the plant's overall size and growth potential. Second, container-grown Marshmallow may require more frequent watering since the soil in containers tends to dry out faster than garden soil. Regular monitoring of soil moisture is essential to prevent the plant from drying out. Additionally, container-grown plants may have different nutrient requirements, as nutrients can be depleted more quickly in containers. Therefore, regular fertilization may be necessary to provide the plant with essential nutrients. Lastly, container-grown Marshmallow may be more susceptible to temperature fluctuations, as the soil in containers can heat up or cool down more quickly compared to the ground. This means that additional protection may be needed during extreme weather conditions to ensure the plant's well-being.

#20 Milkweed – *Asclepias speciosa*

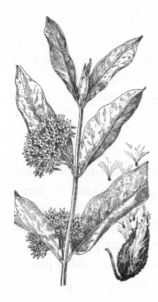

Parts Used: seeds, flowers, roots (leaves used externally only)

Taste: bitter

Actions: cardiotonic, expectorant, anti-tumor, diuretic

Preparation and Dosage: Standard tea dosage applies. Take one teaspoon of the dried flower or root in one cup of boiling water three times daily. Do not use the leaves to make tea. They contain too much oxalic acid.

Common uses: Milkweed is a superior herb for bronchial conditions. It dries up congestion and mucus in the lungs and expels it. It heals gastritis and kidney disorders. Similar to Yellow Dock, it cleanses the blood. The sap heals wounds of all types, even ringworm, and extracts poison from the skin.

Contraindications: Please follow the recommended dosage. The leaves can be toxic if consumed internally. Only use them externally.

Appearance: Perennial plant that typically grows to a height of 2 to 4 feet. It has erect stems with long, lance-shaped leaves arranged in pairs along the stem. The plant produces clusters of small, fragrant flowers in shades of pink, purple, or white. Each flower consists of five petals that curve upward and a central column with a crown of distinctively shaped appendages. As the flowers fade, they are replaced by seed pods that contain numerous seeds attached to silky hairs, which aid in dispersal by wind.

Native Habitat: The native habitat of Milkweed is primarily in the western regions of North America, including parts of the United States and Canada. It is native to areas such as the Rocky Mountains, Great Plains, and western coastal regions.

Planting Milkweed:

Milkweed play a vital role in supporting pollinators, especially monarch butterflies, as milkweed serves as a host plant for their larvae. Milkweed is an important native plant that contributes to the biodiversity and ecological balance of its native habitats.

- **Light:** Milkweed plants prefer full sun and thrive in areas that receive at least 6-8 hours of direct sunlight per day.

- **Watering:** While established Milkweed plants are relatively drought-tolerant, they benefit from regular watering, especially during hot and dry periods. The soil should be kept consistently moist but not waterlogged.

- **Fertilizing:** Milkweed plants generally do not require heavy fertilization.

- **Seasonal adaptability:** Milkweed is a perennial plant that adapts well to different seasons. It goes through growth and flowering in the warmer months and enters dormancy during the colder months.

- **Pruning:** Milkweed plants generally do not require extensive pruning. However, removing spent flowers or cutting back the plant after flowering can help maintain a tidy appearance and promote new growth.

- **Harvesting:**
  - Seeds: Harvest mature pods when they turn brown and begin to split open. Remove the seeds from the pods and separate them from the silky white hairs attached to them.
  - Flowers: Harvest the flowers when they are in full bloom. Carefully pluck the flowers from the plant, ensuring not to damage the delicate structures.
  - Roots: The roots of Milkweed, primarily used for external applications, can also be harvested. Carefully dig around the base of the plant to expose the roots. Extract the desired amount of roots, taking care not to damage the plant.

o   Leaves: Harvest the leaves by carefully plucking them from the plant, ensuring not to damage the stems or other parts of the plant.

Container Gardening:

This plant is primarily grown outdoors in gardens or naturalized areas,

#21 Meadowsweet – *Filipendula ulmaria*

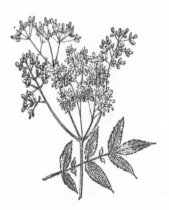

Parts used: aerial parts Temperature: warming

Taste: bitter

Actions: astringent, antacid, anti-emetic, anti-rheumatic, anti-inflammatory, carminative

Preparation and Dosage: Standard Infusion applies; take one teaspoon of the dried herb in one cup of boiling water. Drink three cups daily.

Common uses: It reduces acidity and eases nausea; therefore, it is very calming in the treatment of heartburn. Its astringent quality helps decrease diarrhea. Meadowsweet does contain salicylic acid (the same substance used in aspirin) not as much as in White Willow, but it still can reduce inflammation. It relieves fever, rheumatism, arthritis, and other joint aches.

Contraindications: Please follow the recommended dosage. Meadowsweet is an astringent herb. Drink plenty of water while you take it to rehydrate.

Appearance: Beautiful perennial herb that displays clusters of creamy white or pink flowers atop tall, slender stems. The flowers are complemented by pinnate, fern-like leaves that have a vibrant green color. The plant can reach a height of about 3 to 5 feet and has a bushy growth habit.

Native Habitat: Meadowsweet or Mead Wort is a perennial herb that grows in damp meadows. It is native throughout most of Europe and Western Asia. Now it is commonly grown throughout North America. It is a stately-looking plant that can grow up to 5 ft tall. The dark brown stems are thick and crowned with a tip spray of tiny white flowers in a cone shape.

Planting Meadowsweet:

Meadowsweet is known to attract pollinators, such as bees and butterflies, adding to its appeal for gardeners. It is valued for its ornamental value as well as its traditional medicinal uses.

- **Light:** Meadowsweet thrives in full sun to partial shade. It prefers at least 6 hours of direct sunlight per day, but it can tolerate some shade.

- **Watering:** Meadowsweet requires consistent moisture, especially during the growing season. Keep the soil evenly moist, but avoid overwatering or allowing the soil to become waterlogged.

- **Fertilizing:** Meadowsweet typically doesn't require heavy fertilization. You can apply a balanced organic fertilizer in early spring to promote healthy growth.

- **Seasonal adaptability:** Meadowsweet is a hardy perennial plant that adapts well to different climates. It is generally tolerant of colder temperatures and can be grown in various regions.

- **Pruning:** Prune meadowsweet in early spring before new growth appears. Remove any dead or damaged stems, and thin out overcrowded areas to improve airflow and prevent diseases.

- **Harvesting:** The flowers of meadowsweet are typically harvested in the summer when they are fully open. Cut the flowering stems at the base, taking care not to damage the plant. The flowers can be used fresh or dried for herbal preparations, such as teas or tinctures. The leaves can also be harvested throughout the growing season, but they are best when collected before the plant flowers.

Container Gardening:

While Meadowsweet is commonly cultivated in gardens and naturalized areas, it is not as commonly grown in containers. Meadowsweet is a perennial herb that prefers moist soil and can grow quite tall, making it more suitable for open garden spaces.

#22 Mint – *Mentha piperita*

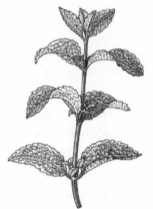

Parts used: aerial parts

Taste: aromatic, slightly bitter

Actions: nervine, antimicrobial, analgesic, aromatic, anti-inflammatory, carminative, diaphoretic, antiemetic, biliary

Preparation and Dosage: Make a Standard Infusion with one teaspoon of the dried herb per cup of boiling water. Drink three cups daily.

Common uses: It is a wonderful carminative; it relaxes the spasms in the digestive system's muscles; it can also assist with flatulence. It relieves intestinal colic, dyspepsia, and similar conditions. Peppermint or any Mint can ease nausea during pregnancy or travel sickness. Peppermint can treat ulcerations in the bowels. It can help in a state of lethargy or lack of concentration.

Contraindications: Mint is safe. Follow the recommended dosage.

Appearance: Mint plants can vary in size, ranging from compact varieties that grow about 6-12 inches tall to larger varieties that can reach up to 3 feet in height. It is a perennial herb that grows in a clumping habit. It has square-shaped stems that are typically green, although some varieties may have reddish or purple hues. The leaves of mint are small, oval-shaped, and have a slightly fuzzy texture.

Native Habitat: Mint is native to Europe and Asia but has naturalized in many other regions around the world.

Planting Mint:

Mint plants have a tendency to grow and spread quickly. They can produce runners or underground stems called rhizomes, which allow them to spread horizontally and create a dense carpet of foliage. This rapid growth and spreading habit make mint plants excellent ground covers or fillers in garden beds. However, it's important to note that this vigorous growth can also make mint plants invasive if not properly contained or managed.

- **Light:** Mint prefers full sun to partial shade. It thrives in bright, indirect light.

- **Watering:** Mint requires regular watering to keep the soil consistently moist. Avoid overwatering or allowing the soil to become waterlogged.

- **Fertilizing:** Mint benefits from regular fertilization to promote healthy growth. Apply a balanced, water-soluble fertilizer according to the manufacturer's instructions during the growing season.

- **Seasonal adaptability:** Mint is a hardy plant that adapts well to different seasons. It is typically grown as an annual but can also be grown as a perennial in suitable climates.

- **Pruning:** Pruning mint regularly helps to control its growth and maintain a compact shape. Pinch off the top few inches of the stems to encourage branching and bushier growth.

- **Harvesting:** Mint leaves can be harvested at any time during the growing season. Harvest by cutting the stems just above a set of leaves. For the best flavor, harvest mint leaves before the plant flowers.

Container Gardening:

Container-grown mint may require more frequent watering and fertilization compared to outdoor gardening due to the limited soil volume and potential for quicker drying. Proper drainage and regular maintenance are essential to ensure the best growing conditions for mint in containers.

Mint plants have a vigorous growth habit and can quickly fill up the available space in a container, potentially leading to issues such as root congestion. To prevent this, it is recommended to periodically divide and repot the mint plant to provide enough space for the roots to grow. Another option is to prune the roots to keep them in check. Regular monitoring of root growth and providing adequate space will help maintain a healthy mint plant and prevent problems associated with root congestion.

#23 Mugwort – *Artemisia vulgaris*

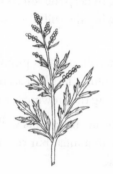

Parts used: leaves

Taste: bitter, acrid

Actions: anthelmintic, vermifuge, diaphoretic, mild narcotic, oxytocic

Preparation and Dosage: Make a Standard Infusion with one teaspoon of the dried herb in 1 cup of boiling water. Take 3 cups daily.

Common uses: Mugwort tincture treats the stomach and intestinal problems and helps with digestion. It is an excellent remedy for worms. It is also a noteworthy herb for controlling shaking induced by nervousness or insomnia. Mugwort is an *extremely bitter* herb. Mugwort is applied topically in a poultice or taken as tea internally to stop hemorrhaging or bleeding. Poultices from the leaves serve to heal wounds.

Contraindications: Avoid using during pregnancy.

Appearance: Herbaceous perennial plant that typically reaches a height of 2 to 4 feet. It has deeply lobed, dark green leaves with a silver-gray underside, giving it a two-toned appearance. The leaves are typically aromatic when crushed, emitting a strong, pleasant fragrance. Mugwort produces tall, upright stems with small, inconspicuous flowers that are greenish-yellow in color. The plant has a bushy and slightly spreading growth habit, forming dense clumps.

Native Habitat: *Artemisia vulgaris* proliferates in high-elevation pastures, forest edges, valleys, hillside wastelands, ditches, and roadsides. The stems are branched and purplish brown. The ascending stems have short hairs. The lobed leaf version is widespread in the Northeast. It has medium-sized lobed leaves that are dark green on the top and papery white underneath.

Planting Mugwort:

Mugwort adds texture and visual interest to your garden, especially with its silver-green leaves and tall, upright growth. It also attracts beneficial insects and pollinators to your garden, making it a valuable addition for biodiversity.

- **Soil:** Mugwort prefers well-drained, loamy soil. It can tolerate poor soils but performs best in fertile soil with good moisture retention.

- **Watering:** Mugwort prefers moist soil and should be watered regularly, especially during dry periods. However, be cautious not to overwater, as it can be susceptible to root rot.

- **Fertilizing:** Mugwort generally doesn't require heavy fertilization. A moderate application of balanced organic fertilizer in spring can be beneficial.

- **Seasonal adaptability:** Mugwort is a hardy perennial that adapts well to various seasons. It can tolerate both sun and partial shade.

- **Pruning:** Pruning is not typically necessary for Mugwort. However, you can trim back any excessive growth or spent flower stalks to maintain a tidy appearance.

- **Harvesting:** Harvest the leaves and flowering tops of Mugwort when they are at their peak potency. It is best to harvest in the morning after the dew has dried but before the sun is at its strongest.

Container Gardening:

Mugwort is not commonly planted in containers due to its spreading growth habit and larger size. It tends to thrive better in open garden spaces where it has room to spread and grow to its full potential.

#24 Mullein – *Verbascum thapsus*

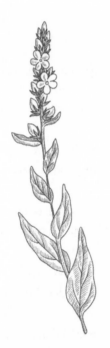

Parts used: leaf, flower and root

Taste: slightly bitter

Actions: expectorant, demulcent, antitussive, astringent, and vulnerary

Preparation and Dosage: Make a Standard Infusion with one teaspoon of the dried leaves or flowers in 1 cup of boiling water. Take three cups daily.

Common uses: You could call this herb the ideal family herb. Mullein is for bronchial and lung congestion; it is a gentle enough herb for children and the elderly. Often, it can ease lymphatic congestion. It is effective in dry, irritated bronchial tissues resulting from a consistent dry hacking cough, a respiratory infection, or smoking. It was a traditional remedy for tuberculosis and could calm the coughing spasms of the lungs.

Mullein ear oil, found in the recipe section, is effective for throbbing in the ear or pain from an ear infection.

Contraindications: Please follow the recommended dosage.

Appearance: Biennial plant that varies in size throughout its lifecycle. In its first year, it forms a low-growing rosette of large, fuzzy leaves that can reach a diameter of 1 to 2 feet. These leaves are gray-green in color and have an oblong or lance-shaped appearance. In the second year,

Mullein sends up a tall flower stalk that can reach impressive heights of 6 feet or more. The flower spike is adorned with numerous small, yellow flowers arranged in a dense, cylindrical cluster. The flowers bloom from the bottom to the top, creating a visually stunning display.

Native Habitat: Mullein is a biennial, striking plant that comes from Europe. It sends an impressive yellow floral spike up through a silvery green base of leaves. This plant grows on roadsides, sunlit gravel, or sandy areas.

Planting Mullein:

The combination of the large rosette of leaves and the tall flower spike makes Mullein a distinct and eye-catching plant in the garden.

- **Planting:** Mullein is typically grown from seeds, which can be sown directly into the garden soil or started indoors and transplanted later.

- **Soil:** Mullein thrives in well-drained soil, including sandy or rocky soil. It can adapt to different soil types, including poor or dry soils.

- **Watering:** Mullein prefers well-drained soil and can tolerate dry conditions. Water moderately, allowing the soil to dry out slightly between waterings.

- **Fertilizing:** Mullein doesn't require fertilization.

- **Seasonal adaptability:** Mullein is a biennial plant that can adapt to different seasons. It prefers full sun but can tolerate partial shade.

- **Pruning:** Pruning is generally not necessary for Mullein. However, you can remove spent flower stalks to encourage new growth and extend the blooming period.

- **Harvesting:** Harvest the leaves and flowers of Mullein when they are fully developed but before they begin to wilt. Handle the leaves with care, as they are delicate and can easily break.

Container Gardening:

While Mullein is primarily grown in gardens, it can also be successfully cultivated in containers. Growing Mullein in containers allows for better control over its size and spread, making it suitable for smaller spaces or urban gardening. Choose a large container with good drainage and fill it with well-draining potting soil. Place the container in a sunny location, as Mullein thrives in full sun. Regular watering is essential to keep the soil evenly moist, but avoid overwatering, as Mullein prefers slightly drier conditions. Fertilize the plant with a balanced fertilizer once a month during the growing season to promote healthy growth. Pruning is generally not necessary unless you want to control its size or remove spent flower stalks.

#25 Nettle – *Urtica dioica*

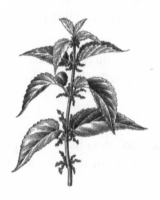

Parts Used: leaves

Taste: bitter

Actions: detoxification, tonic, antihistamine, immunostimulating, adaptogenic, expectorant, oxytocic

Preparation and Dosage: Standard tea dosage applies. Take one teaspoon of the dried leaf in one cup of boiling water three times daily. Or, if you have access to the fresh leaves, cook them like spinach and take 2 oz to 4 oz a few times a week.

Common uses: Nettles are both a superfood and a full-spectrum herb. They are incredibly high in minerals, calcium, magnesium, potassium, iron, phosphorus, manganese, and silica. They are an excellent source of vitamin C, B vitamins, and chlorophyll. Nettles are perfect for immune support and reduce most allergic responses. They restore kidney and liver function, build blood and alleviate anemia. If a person is weak from illness or chronically sick from any ailment, Nettle is a great recovery herb.

Contraindications: Please follow the recommended dosage. Nettles are a strong detoxifying herb. Detoxifying too quickly or without drinking enough water may cause a headache.

Appearance: Nettle plants vary in size, with some growing as tall as 2 to 4 feet, while others can reach up to 7 feet in height. This perennial herb has erected, square-shaped stems covered in fine hairs, and the stems are usually green with a slightly reddish tint. The leaves are lance-shaped, toothed, and covered in tiny stinging hairs.

Native Habitat: Native to Europe, Asia, and North Africa.

Planting Nettle:

Nettle can be an aggressive spreader, so it's recommended to plant it in a contained area or in a pot to prevent it from taking over the garden. However, Nettle is a valuable addition to your garden, serving multiple purposes. It acts as a natural pest deterrent, repelling insects like aphids and whiteflies, making it an excellent companion plant for vulnerable crops. Nettles also attract beneficial insects such as ladybugs and lacewings, which help control garden pests. Additionally, Nettles deep roots allow it to absorb and accumulate nutrients, particularly nitrogen, making it a nutrient accumulator. You can harvest nettle leaves to use as a nutrient-rich mulch or make nettle tea as a natural fertilizer for other plants. Adding nettles to your compost pile can enhance its nutrient content and decomposition process. By incorporating nettle strategically in your garden, you can benefit from its pest control properties, nutrient accumulation, and support for beneficial insects.

- **Soil:** Nettle prefers rich, moist soil with good drainage. It can tolerate a range of soil types but thrives in fertile soils.

- **Watering:** Keep the soil consistently moist, especially during dry periods. Avoid overwatering to prevent waterlogged conditions.

- **Fertilizing:** Nettle is a nutrient accumulator and typically does not require additional fertilization. However, if the soil is poor, you can supplement with organic compost or a balanced fertilizer during the growing season.

- **Seasonal adaptability:** Nettle is a perennial plant that adapts well to different seasons. It can tolerate both cool and warm temperatures and is known for its resilience.

- **Pruning:** Pruning nettle is not necessary unless you want to control its spread. If desired, you can trim back the plant in early spring to encourage bushier growth.

- **Harvesting:** Harvest nettle leaves when they are young and tender, typically in spring or early summer. Wear protective gloves to avoid stinging. Cut the top portion of the plant or use scissors to snip off individual leaves. Harvesting should be done before the plant flowers for the best flavor and quality.

Container Gardening:

It's not very common to plant Nettle in pots.

#26 Oregano – *Origanum vulgare*

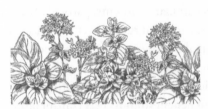

Parts used: aerial parts

Taste: aromatic, slightly bitter

Actions: anti-inflammatory, carminative hepatics, anti-spasmodic (digestion)

Preparation and Dosage: Prepare a Standard Infusion by steeping one teaspoon of dried herb in a cup of boiling water. Drink three cups daily.

Common uses: Culinary herb used for cooking. Oregano, a member of the mint family, shares many benefits with other mint varieties. It is particularly known for its carminative properties, helping to relax digestive spasms and relieve conditions such as flatulence, intestinal colic, and an upset stomach. Oregano can also be used to alleviate nausea during pregnancy or travel sickness.

Contraindications: Oregano is generally safe when used in recommended dosages. However, avoid using it as a medicine during pregnancy and if you have a gallbladder or liver disease. External use may cause skin irritation. Not recommended for children under the age of two.

Appearance: Oregano plants vary in size, with compact varieties reaching about 6-12 inches in height and larger varieties growing up to 3 feet tall. This perennial herb grows in clumps and has square-shaped stems that are typically green, sometimes with reddish or purple hues. The leaves are small, oval-shaped, and slightly fuzzy.

Native Habitat: Oregano is native to Europe and Asia but has naturalized in various regions worldwide.

Planting Oregano:

Oregano is commonly grown in gardens for its aromatic leaves that are used in various Mediterranean and Italian dishes. It is often used fresh or dried to enhance the flavors of pizzas, pasta sauces, salads, and more. It is easy to cultivate and maintain.

- **Soil:** Oregano thrives in well-draining soil that is moderately fertile. A loamy or sandy soil with a pH level around 6.0 to 8.0 is suitable for its growth.

- **Light:** Oregano prefers full sun, although it can tolerate partial shade. It requires at least 6 hours of direct sunlight per day for optimal growth and flavor development.

- **Watering:** Oregano is drought-tolerant and prefers to be on the drier side. Water the plant deeply but infrequently, allowing the soil to dry out between waterings.

- **Fertilizing:** Oregano doesn't require heavy fertilization. You can amend the soil with organic matter before planting, and a light application of balanced fertilizer in early spring can provide additional nutrients.

- **Seasonal adaptability:** Oregano is a perennial herb that is hardy in USDA zones 4-9. It can tolerate a wide range of temperatures and is best suited for moderate climates. It may go dormant or die back in colder regions during winter.

- **Pruning:** Regular pruning of oregano helps to maintain its shape, promote bushier growth, and prevent it from becoming woody. Trim back the stems by one-third in early spring or after flowering.

- **Harvesting:** Oregano leaves can be harvested as needed once the plant reaches a height of about 4-6 inches. Harvest the outer leaves by snipping them close to the stem. For the best flavor, harvest before the plant starts to flower.

Container Gardening:

Container-grown oregano can be easily moved indoors during colder months or placed on patios, balconies, or windowsills for convenient access to fresh herbs. It is important to choose a well-draining container and provide adequate sunlight and watering for optimal growth.

#27 Parsley – Petroselinum crispum

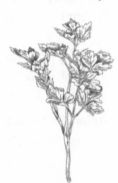

Parts used: leaves, stems, roots (less common)

Attention: the plant known as 'parsley root' is also called 'Hamburg root' and is another plant. Parsley root, derived from the subspecies of garden parsley scientifically known as *Petroselinum crispum Tuberosum*, is primarily cultivated for its thick and tuberous roots.

Taste: fresh, slightly bitter, aromatic

UNLOCK THE SECRETS OF PLANT MEDICINE AT HOME

Actions: emmenagogue, diuretic, carminative

Preparation and Dosage: Use fresh or dried parsley leaves as a culinary herb in various dishes. As a medicinal herb, prepare a tea by steeping 1-2 teaspoons of dried parsley leaves in a cup of hot water for 5-10 minutes. Drink up to three cups daily.

Common uses: Parsley is commonly used as a culinary herb to enhance the flavor of dishes. Medicinally, it is known for its diuretic properties, promoting urine production and aiding in detoxification. It acts as a carminative, helping to relieve digestive discomfort and reduce bloating and gas. Parsley is considered a digestive tonic, supporting healthy digestion and promoting nutrient absorption. It possesses antioxidant properties, protecting the body against oxidative stress. It also exhibits antimicrobial activity against certain bacteria and fungi.

Parsley has been traditionally used as an emmenagogue in herbal medicine to help regulate menstruation and promote menstrual flow.

Contraindications: Large amounts of parsley should be avoided during pregnancy, as it may stimulate the uterus. Some individuals may have allergic reactions to parsley, so caution should be exercised if you have known allergies to other plants in the Apiaceae family.

Appearance: Parsley is a biennial herb that typically grows up to 1-2 feet in height. It has bright green, flat or curly leaves that grow in a rosette pattern. The plant produces small, greenish-yellow flowers in umbels, which later develop into seeds known as parsley seeds.

Native Habitat: Parsley is native to the Mediterranean region but is now cultivated in many parts of the world. It prefers well-drained soil and full sun or partial shade.

Planting Parsley:

Both flat-leaf parsley and curly parsley belong to the same species, *Petroselinum crispum*, and share similar medicinal properties. Flat-leaf parsley tends to be more popular among home gardeners and culinary enthusiasts due to its stronger flavor and preferred culinary uses. Its broader leaves are often favored for cooking and garnishing dishes. Curly parsley, with its attractive ruffled leaves, is also grown but is generally regarded as more decorative rather than primarily used for culinary purposes.

- **Soil:** Parsley prefers well-draining soil that is rich in organic matter. A loamy soil with a slightly acidic to neutral pH is ideal for its growth.

- **Light:** Parsley thrives in full sun to partial shade. It requires at least 4-6 hours of direct sunlight per day for optimal growth.

- **Watering:** Keep the soil consistently moist but not waterlogged. Water parsley regularly, especially during dry periods, and ensure the soil remains evenly moist.

- **Fertilizing:** Apply a balanced fertilizer or compost to the soil before planting. Additionally, you can feed parsley with a diluted liquid fertilizer every 4-6 weeks during the growing season.

- **Seasonal adaptability:** Parsley is a cool-season herb that can tolerate light frosts. It is typically grown as an annual but can sometimes survive as a biennial. It thrives in mild temperatures and may bolt and go to seed in hot summer weather.

- **Pruning:** Regularly harvest parsley leaves to encourage bushier growth. Pinch or trim off the outer stems or leaves as needed, leaving the inner leaves to continue growing.

- **Harvesting:** You can start harvesting parsley leaves when the plant has developed enough foliage. Harvest the outer leaves by cutting them close to the base of the plant, leaving the inner leaves to continue growing. You can harvest parsley throughout the growing season as needed.

Container Gardening:

Parsley is popularly grown in both gardens and containers. When planted in containers, parsley requires a well-draining potting mix. Choose a container with good drainage holes and provide adequate sunlight or partial shade. Water regularly to keep the soil consistently moist.

Container-grown parsley may require more frequent fertilization to provide essential nutrients. Prune regularly to promote bushier growth and harvest leaves as needed. Ensure the container is large enough to accommodate the root system of parsley.

#28 Passionflower – *Passiflora incarnata*

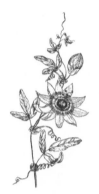

Parts used: aerial parts (leaves, stems, flowers)

Taste: slightly bitter, earthy

Actions: anti-inflammatory, antispasmodic, antitussive, hypotensive and sedative

Preparation and Dosage: Prepare a standard infusion by steeping 1-2 teaspoons of the dried passionflower in a cup of boiling water. Steep for 10 minutes. Drink up to three cups daily.

Common uses: Passionflower is known for its sedative and anxiolytic properties, making it useful for reducing anxiety, promoting relaxation, and improving sleep quality. It is also a powerful nervine, helping to calm the nervous system and relieve nervous tension. Passionflower can be used for its antispasmodic effects to alleviate muscle spasms and cramps. Additionally, it has hypotensive properties and may help lower blood pressure.

Contraindications: Since passionflower appears to act on the central nervous system it should not be taken by people already using antidepressants, sedative medication or during pregnancy.

Appearance: Passionflower is a vine-like plant that can grow up to 30 feet in length. It has lobed leaves and intricate, showy flowers with a unique structure. The flowers are typically white with purple or blue accents. The plant produces small, round, orange-yellow fruits.

Native Habitat: Passionflower is native to the southeastern United States but has naturalized in other regions with similar climates.

Planting Passionflower:

One of the reasons why passionflower is popular is its unique and beautiful blooms. They can add a touch of elegance and tropical flair to garden landscapes, attracting butterflies and hummingbirds.

- **Soil:** Passionflower prefers well-draining soil that is rich in organic matter. A loamy or sandy soil with a slightly acidic to neutral pH is ideal for its growth.

- **Light:** Passionflower thrives in full sun to partial shade. It requires at least 6-8 hours of direct sunlight per day for optimal growth and flowering.

- **Watering:** Keep the soil consistently moist but not waterlogged. Water passionflower regularly, especially during dry periods, and ensure the soil remains evenly moist.

- **Fertilizing:** Apply a balanced fertilizer or organic compost to the soil before planting. Additionally, you can provide supplemental fertilization during the growing season with a slow-release or liquid fertilizer, following the package instructions.

- **Seasonal adaptability:** Passionflower is a perennial vine that is hardy in USDA zones 6-9. It prefers warm temperatures and may go dormant or die back in colder regions. Provide protection or bring potted plants indoors during frost or freezing conditions.

- **Pruning:** Prune passionflower in early spring to remove dead or damaged growth and shape the plant. You can also prune lightly throughout the growing season to control its size and encourage branching.

- **Harvesting:** Harvest passionflower aerial parts, such as leaves, flowers, and stems, when they are fully mature and at their peak potency. Gently pluck or cut the desired parts from the plant, taking care not to damage the rest of the plant. Use harvested parts immediately or dry them for later use.

Container Gardening:

When planted in containers, passion flowers have restricted root growth and limited space, which can result in smaller plant size and reduced spread. When planting passion flowers in containers, there are a few considerations to keep in mind. Firstly, choose a container that is large enough to accommodate the plant's root system and provide adequate drainage. Use a well-draining potting mix specifically formulated for container gardening. Regular watering is crucial for container plants, as they can dry out more quickly than those planted in the ground. Fertilize the plant regularly with a balanced fertilizer to ensure it receives necessary nutrients. Additionally, container-grown passion flowers may benefit from occasional pruning to maintain their size and shape.

#29 Plantain – *Plantago major*

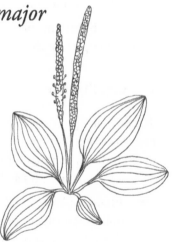

Parts Used: leaves or aerial parts Temperature: cooling

Taste: slightly bitter

Actions: anesthetic, vulnerary, expectorant, demulcent, anti-inflammatory, astringent, diuretic, antimicrobial

Preparation and Dosage:

1. Take one teaspoon of the dried herb in 1 cup of boiling water three times daily.

2. Make a poultice by macerating two tablespoons of the leaves. Add one teaspoon of water.

3. Wash the leaves and add them to salads.

Common uses: The wide-leaf Plantain and its close relative Ribwort Plantain have valuable healing properties. Its power to extract toxins, poisons, and even small objects from the skin is remarkable. Plantain acts as a gentle expectorant. Its soothing, demulcent quality is perfect for inflamed and sore membranes. It works as a respiratory herb and can help soothe coughs and milder cases of bronchitis. It is ideal for children and more vulnerable populations. Its astringent qualities can help with diarrhea and hemorrhoids.

Contraindications: This gentle herb is very safe for children and the elderly. Please follow the recommended dosage.

Appearance: There are about 200 species in the Plantago genus. The three most common varieties found in the US are broadleaf plantain (*P. major*), Rugel's plantain (*P. rugelii*), and ribwort plantain (*P. lanceolata*). Plantago consists of broad leaves with equal parted leaves that fan out in groups or basal rosettes from the low base of the plant. The other variety, Ribwort, or long-leaved plantain has long, thin and very prominent ribbed leaves that rise up from the base. Both plants have a long stalk with seedlings that come up from the middle.

Native Habitat: This plant is native to Europe and has naturalized in many other parts of the world, including North America.

Planting Plantain:

Typically, not grown as such in gardens or containers but is very easy to find. Look for Plantain in vacant lots and waste areas or sunny meadows. However, you may also want to plant it in your garden but . Just be sure to contain it. It's an invasive plant.

- **Planting:** You can get the seeds from wild plants or order them online. An easier option is to find wild plantain and transplant them directly into your garden.

- **Soil:** Plantain is adaptable to a wide range of soil types, but it prefers well-draining soil. Loamy or sandy soil with a slightly acidic to neutral pH is ideal for its growth.

- **Light:** Plantain can tolerate various light conditions but thrives in full sun to partial shade. It can grow in both shaded and sunny areas of the garden.

- **Watering:** Plantain requires regular watering to keep the soil consistently moist. However, it is important not to overwater, as excessive moisture can lead to root rot. Water the plants deeply but allow the soil to dry slightly between waterings.

- **Fertilizing:** Plantain generally does not require heavy fertilization.

- **Seasonal adaptability:** Plantain is a hardy perennial herb that adapts well to different seasons. It can withstand both cold and hot temperatures, making it suitable for various climates. It typically grows and flourishes during the spring and summer months.

- **Pruning:** Pruning is not necessary for Plantain, as it naturally forms a rosette of leaves close to the ground. However, you can remove any damaged or yellowing leaves as needed to maintain the plant's appearance and health.

- **Harvesting:** Plantain leaves can be harvested throughout the growing season. Select mature leaves and gently pluck or cut them near the base of the plant. It is best to harvest the leaves in the morning when their medicinal properties are most potent. You can use the fresh leaves immediately or dry them for future use.

Container Gardening:

The main difference when planting Plantain in pots compared to garden beds is the limited space and root confinement. Potted Plantain has restricted root growth and may require more frequent watering and fertilizing to meet its nutrient needs. Additionally, container-grown Plantain may be more susceptible to temperature fluctuations, requiring extra care to protect them from extreme heat or cold.

#30 Red Clover – *Trifolium pratense*

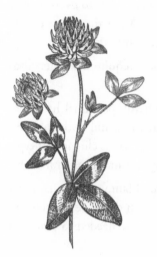

Parts Used: flower

Taste: aromatic, slightly bitter

Actions: alterative, expectorant

Preparation and Dosage: Make a Standard Infusion of the dried flowers with 1½ teaspoons of the dried flower per 1 cup of boiling water. Take 3 cups daily.

Common uses: Red Clover is one of the most valuable remedies for children's skin problems. It detoxifies the blood. When toxins are flushed out of the blood in general skin conditions often improve.

Its expectorant actions make this remedy useful when treating coughs and bronchitis. It even treats whooping cough. It is effective when combined with other herbs to treat anemia. Europeans introduced this herb to the Americas.

Contraindications: Please follow the recommended dosage.

Appearance: Herbaceous perennial plant that typically grows to a height of 1 to 2 feet. It has a dense, rounded growth habit with multiple stems arising from a central crown. The leaves are alternate, trifoliate, and oval-shaped with serrated edges. The vibrant pink to purple flowers are arranged in dense, cylindrical clusters at the top of the stems. Each flower is composed of numerous tiny florets. The plant has a deep taproot system and may develop runners that allow it to spread.

Native Habitat: Native to Europe, Western Asia, and Northwest Africa.

Planting Red Clover:

There are several reasons why you might consider planting red clover in your garden. First and foremost, red clover is a beneficial plant for pollinators, attracting bees and other beneficial insects to your garden.

It also helps to improve soil health by fixing nitrogen from the atmosphere into the soil, enriching it with this essential nutrient. Red clover can act as a natural ground cover, suppressing weed growth and preventing erosion.

- **Soil:** Red clover prefers well-drained soil that is fertile and loamy. It can tolerate a wide range of soil pH, but a slightly acidic to neutral pH is ideal for its growth.

- **Light:** Red clover thrives in full sun to partial shade. It requires at least 4-6 hours of direct sunlight per day for optimal growth and flowering.

- **Watering:** Keep the soil consistently moist, especially during dry periods. Water red clover regularly, aiming to keep the soil evenly moist but not waterlogged.

- **Fertilizing:** Red clover is a legume that can fix nitrogen from the atmosphere, reducing the need for additional fertilization. However, if the soil is nutrient-poor, you can apply a balanced organic fertilizer before planting.

- **Seasonal adaptability:** Red clover is a cool-season perennial that can tolerate cold temperatures. It grows best in moderate climates but can also tolerate some heat. It may die back during hot summers or in regions with extremely cold winters.

- **Pruning:** Red clover doesn't require pruning, but you can mow or cut it back after flowering to promote fresh growth and prevent self-seeding if desired.

- **Harvesting:** The aerial parts of the plant, including the leaves and flowers, are typically harvested when the plant is in full bloom. This is when the concentration of beneficial compounds is at its highest. Harvesting can be done by cutting the plant near the base, leaving some stem length for drying or processing.

Container Gardening:

Red Clover is not commonly grown in containers.

#31 Roses and Rosehips – *Rosa canina*

Parts Used: flower and rosehip.

Temperature: cooling

Taste: flower is aromatic, rosehips are sour and astringent

Actions:

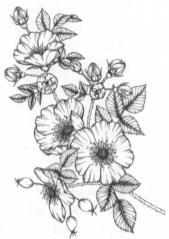

- **Rose:** anti-inflammatory, adaptogenic, diaphoretic, anti-microbial, cardiotonic

- **Rosehips:** nutritive, adaptogenic, astringent, tonic, vulnerary, anti-inflammatory

Preparation and Dosage: Rose petals do not make a good solitary tincture. They are too delicate, and the alcohol in the tincture diminishes the smell, its primary benefit. Rose is mild, so make an infusion with one tablespoon of the fresh petals per cup of boiling water or a rounded teaspoon of the dried. Take one cup three times daily. For Rosehip tea, put one teaspoon of the dried fruit in 1 cup of boiling water. Take three cups daily.

Common uses: Rose is an ideal remedy for grief, shock, and trauma. It shifts someone from a mild or deep depression to an uplifted state.

Contraindications: Both Rose and Rosehips are mild herbs with no known side effects.

Appearance: Roses are deciduous shrubs that can vary in size depending on the cultivar. They typically grow between 3 to 6 feet in height, but some varieties can reach up to 20 feet. They have thorny stems and pinnate leaves with serrated edges. The flowers of roses come in various colors, including shades of red, pink, yellow, white, and orange.

Many people have a Rosebush in their yard and yet are unaware that after the Rose fades away, a marvelous reddish bulb appears in its place that has excellent medicinal value.

Rosehips contain 4% vitamin C. The synergistic components of Rosehips maximize Vitamin C absorption. Rosehips scavenge free radicals with their antioxidant capabilities. They are anti-inflammatory, stabilize collagen, and help heal wounds and have been known to reduce tumors. Rosehips elevate the white blood cell count, enhancing immunity.

Native Habitat: *Rosa canina*, commonly known as wild rose or dog rose, is native to Europe, North Africa, and Asia. It is a hardy plant that can thrive in a variety of habitats, including woodlands, meadows, and hedgerows.

Planting Roses:

The decision to grow roses in gardens or containers depends on individual preferences and the available space. While roses can be rewarding with their beauty and the harvest of rosehips, they require diligent care and attention to thrive.

- **Soil:** Prefers well-draining soil that is rich in organic matter. A loamy soil with a slightly acidic to neutral pH is suitable for its growth.

- **Light:** Thrive in full sun but can tolerate partial shade. They require at least 6-8 hours of direct sunlight per day for optimal growth and flowering.

- **Watering:** Keep the soil consistently moist but not waterlogged. Water deeply at the base of the plant to encourage deep root growth. Avoid overhead watering, as it can lead to fungal diseases.

- **Fertilizing:** Apply a balanced rose fertilizer or organic compost in early spring to provide essential nutrients for healthy growth and blooming.

- **Seasonal adaptability:** Rosa canina is a hardy plant that can tolerate various seasonal conditions. It is adaptable to both cool and warm climates.

- **Pruning:** Regular pruning helps maintain the shape and health of the plant. Prune in late winter or early spring to remove dead or weak wood and promote new growth.

- **Harvesting:** Rosa canina produces rosehips, which can be harvested in late summer or early autumn when they are fully ripened and have turned vibrant red or orange. Harvest by cutting or gently twisting the rosehips from the stems.

Container Gardening:

While roses can be successfully grown in containers, there are some considerations to keep in mind. Container-grown roses require larger containers with good drainage and a high-quality potting mix. They need consistent watering, as containers can dry out more quickly than garden soil. Regular fertilization is also necessary to provide the necessary nutrients. Pruning should be done to control size and shape, as well as to promote air circulation.

#32 Rosemary – *Rosemarinus officinalis*

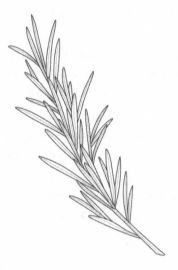

Parts Used: Leaves and stems

Temperature: warming

Taste: aromatic, bitter, pungent

Actions: adaptogenic, anti-inflammatory, carminative, rubefacient, hepatoprotective, stimulates hair growth, improves memory, cephalic (relates to the head), oxytocic

Preparation and Dosage: Make a Standard Infusion. Take one teaspoon of the dried herb in 1 cup of boiling water three times daily.

Common uses: Rosemary is a stimulant for the circulatory system. It is warm and pungent, brings blood to the skin's surface and is helpful for musculoskeletal and neurological pain. Rosemary is an essential herb because it can alleviate mental and physical distress. Its combination of attributes makes it a wonderful cardiotonic herb in cases of weakness and fragility. Rosemary will calm and tone the digestive system, particularly a cranky digestive system that suffers from nervous debilitation.

Contraindications: Please follow the recommended dosage. This herb is hypertensive and might raise blood pressure. Please use it with caution if you have a long and severe history of high blood pressure.

Appearance: Rosemary is an evergreen shrub that grows upright with a dense, bushy habit. It typically reaches a height of about 2 to 4 feet and has a spread of 3 to 4 feet. The plant features needle-like leaves that are dark green on top and grayish-green underneath. The leaves are aromatic and have a resinous fragrance. Rosemary produces small, blue or purple flowers that grow in clusters along the stems. The plant has a woody stem and branches, and it can develop a slightly gnarled and twisted appearance with age.

Native Habitat: The name Rosemary comes from the Latin word Ros Marinus meaning "the rose of the sea." It has an ancient Mediterranean origin. You will recognize it by its unmistakable aroma. You can identify its needles, resembling a miniature version of green balsam fir trees.

Planting Rosemary:

As rosemary is an herb that is easy to grow and low maintenance it can be found in many herb gardens. Its pleasant fragrance can also deter certain pests in the garden, making it a beneficial companion plant.

- **Soil:** Rosemary thrives in well-draining soil that is sandy or loamy. It prefers a slightly acidic to neutral pH level.

- **Light:** Rosemary requires full sun and thrives in hot and sunny conditions. It needs at least 6-8 hours of direct sunlight per day for optimal growth.

- **Watering:** Rosemary prefers dry to moderately moist soil. It is drought-tolerant and should be watered sparingly, allowing the soil to dry out between waterings.

- **Fertilizing:** Rosemary is a low-maintenance herb that doesn't require much fertilization.

- **Seasonal adaptability:** Rosemary is an evergreen perennial that is best suited for warm climates. It can tolerate mild winter temperatures but may require protection or be grown in containers in colder regions.

- **Pruning:** Regular pruning is beneficial for rosemary to maintain its shape and encourage bushier growth. Prune lightly after flowering or as needed to remove dead or leggy branches.

- **Harvesting:** You can harvest rosemary sprigs as needed once the plant has reached a suitable size. Cut the stems just above a leaf node to encourage regrowth. Harvest in the morning when the essential oils are most concentrated.

Container Gardening:

When it comes to growing rosemary in containers, it is well suited to growing on balconies or indoor cultivation. However, it's important to choose a container large enough to accommodate the plant's root system and provide sufficient space for growth.

#33 Sage – *Salvia officinalis*

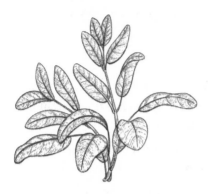

Parts Used: leaves

Taste: aromatic, slightly bitter

Actions: anti-inflammatory, antispasmodic, astringent, carminative, nervine, sedative, oxytocic

Preparation and Dosage: Infuse one teaspoon of the dried herb in 1 cup of boiling water. Just the aroma is a powerful healer for stress.

Common uses: Sage decreases gas, bloating, diarrhea, intestinal spasms, and gastritis.

It is a superior herb for respiratory issues and a classic remedy for a simple sore throat. It acts on the oral cavity and the respiratory system to aid both laryngitis and pharyngitis. You can also use it for bleeding gums by swishing the tea around in your mouth for several minutes.

Sage's aroma assists with depression, anxiety, and mental exhaustion. It is a grounding herb and helps call the user back to the present moment. Much like Rosemary, it increases concentration and memory while decreasing fatigue.

Contraindications: Sage is a gentle herb. Please follow the recommended dosage.

Appearance: Sage is a perennial herb that grows as a compact, bushy plant. It typically reaches a height of about 1 to 2 feet and has a spread of 1 to 2 feet. The plant has long, narrow leaves that are gray-green or silvery in color. The leaves are densely packed on upright stems, giving the plant a full and lush appearance. Sage produces small, tubular flowers that can range in color from purple and blue to white or pink, depending on the variety. The plant has a woody stem and branches, and the leaves have a distinct, savory aroma when crushed.

Native Habitat: Native to the Mediterranean region, specifically to areas in Southern Europe and the Mediterranean basin. It is commonly found in countries such as Greece, Italy, Spain, and Turkey. However, sage has been widely cultivated and naturalized in various parts of the world, including North America, where it is commonly grown as a culinary and medicinal herb.

Planting Sage

Sage is a popular choice for gardeners that appreciate it for its culinary uses, medicinal properties and aesthetic appeal.

- **Soil:** Sage prefers well-draining soil with a pH level between 6.0 and 7.0. Sandy or loamy soil types are ideal for its growth.
- **Light:** Sage requires full sun and thrives in bright, direct sunlight. It needs at least 6-8 hours of sun exposure per day for optimal growth.
- **Watering:** Sage is drought-tolerant and prefers dry to moderately moist soil. Water it sparingly, allowing the soil to dry out between waterings. Overwatering can lead to root rot.
- **Fertilizing:** Sage doesn't require heavy fertilization.
- **Seasonal adaptability:** Sage is a hardy perennial herb that is well-adapted to various climates. It can tolerate hot and dry conditions as well as colder temperatures. It is generally frost-tolerant.
- **Pruning:** Regular pruning helps maintain the shape and vigor of sage plants. Prune lightly after flowering or in early spring to remove any dead or damaged branches.
- **Harvesting:** Sage leaves can be harvested as needed once the plant has become established. Harvest in the morning when the essential oils are most concentrated. Cut the stems just above a leaf node, and avoid removing more than one-third of the plant at a time.

Container Gardening:

Sage plants can be grown in containers of suitable size to accommodate their root system. Choose a container with good drainage to prevent waterlogged soil. The plant's growth may be slightly smaller compared to outdoor plants, but it can still form a compact and attractive bushy shape. Regular pruning can help maintain its shape and size.

#34 St. John's Wort – *Hypericum perforatum*

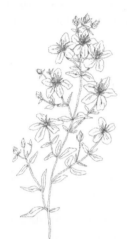

Parts used: aerial parts (flowering tops)

Taste: slightly bitter, astringent

Actions: nervine, anti-inflammatory, analgesic and antiviral

Preparation and Dosage: Prepare an infusion by steeping 1-2 teaspoons of dried herb in a cup of boiling water for 10-15 minutes. Drink up to three cups daily.

Common uses: St. John's Wort is well-known for its antidepressant properties and is often used to alleviate mild to moderate depression and improve mood. It also acts as a nervine, helping to calm the nervous system and reduce anxiety. St. John's Wort has anti-inflammatory and analgesic effects, making it useful for relieving nerve pain and muscle aches. Additionally, it has antiviral properties and may be beneficial for treating viral infections.

St. John's Wort lacks certain side effects commonly seen in prescription antidepressants, such as a decrease in libido. But there is a lack of research on its effects on severe depression so be sure to consult a medic in such a case.

St. Johns's Wort is recognized for its wound healing properties and can be topically applied as infusions or washes to promote the healing of minor wounds, skin sores, and bruises.

Contraindications: St. John's Wort may interact with certain medications, including antidepressants, birth control pills, and blood-thinning medications. Consult with a healthcare professional before using if you are taking any medications. Internal consumption had reports of causing dermatitis or photo sensitivity and being exposed to the sun. Also, contact dermatitis is possible when touching it in moist but sunny conditions.

Appearance: St. John's Wort is a perennial herb with multiple branches that can grow up to 2 feet in height. It has opposite, oblong leaves that are dotted with small, translucent glands. The plant produces bright yellow flowers with five petals and numerous stamens, which bloom from June to September.

Native Habitat: St. John's Wort is native to Europe but has naturalized in many other regions, including North America. It prefers sunny locations and can be found in fields, meadows, and along roadsides.

Planting St. John's Wort:

This is a versatile herb that is popularly grown in gardens in the Midwest.

- **Soil:** St. John's Wort prefers well-draining soil that is fertile and rich in organic matter. A loamy or sandy soil with a pH range of 6.0 to 7.5 is suitable for its growth.

- **Light:** St. John's Wort thrives in full sun to partial shade. It requires at least 6 hours of direct sunlight per day for optimal growth and flowering.

- **Watering:** St. John's Wort is moderately drought-tolerant once established. Water it regularly, providing enough moisture to keep the soil evenly moist but not waterlogged.

- **Fertilizing:** St. John's Wort generally does not require heavy fertilization. However, you can apply a balanced organic fertilizer in early spring to provide some nutrients.

- **Seasonal adaptability:** St. John's Wort is a hardy perennial herb that can adapt to various climates. It can tolerate both warm and cool temperatures and is generally frost-tolerant.

- **Pruning:** Prune St. John's Wort in late winter or early spring to remove dead or damaged branches and promote new growth. It can also benefit from a light pruning after flowering to maintain its shape and encourage bushiness.

- **Harvesting:** Harvest the aerial parts of St. John's Wort, including the flowers and leaves, when the plant is in full bloom. Gather the plant material in dry weather and dry it thoroughly before storage.

Container Gardening:

While growing St. John's Wort in containers is not as common as planting it in gardens, it is still practiced by some gardeners and herbal enthusiasts. Opt for a container with proper drainage to ensure the soil doesn't become waterlogged. Although container-grown plants may be slightly smaller compared to those grown outdoors, they can still develop a compact and attractive bushy form. Regular pruning will help maintain the plant's shape and size.

#35 Thyme – *Thymus vulgaris*

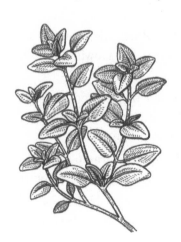

Parts used: leaves, flowers

Taste: aromatic, slightly pungent

Actions: expectorant, carminative

Preparation and Dosage: Infuse 1-2 teaspoons of dried thyme in a cup of boiling water for 10 minutes. Strain and drink up to three cups per day.

Common uses: Culinary herb for example fitting to fish, meat, and vegetables. Thyme is valued for its antimicrobial properties and is often used to treat respiratory infections, coughs, and congestion. It acts as an expectorant, helping to loosen and expel mucus from the lungs. Thyme also has antispasmodic properties that can provide relief from spasms in the digestive system, reducing symptoms of indigestion and flatulence. It is a carminative herb, aiding digestion and alleviating bloating. Thyme is known for its antioxidant properties, which help protect the body against oxidative stress. It has diuretic effects, promoting urine production and supporting kidney health.

Contraindications: Avoid using thyme in large amounts during pregnancy. It may cause allergic reactions in individuals sensitive to the *Lamiaceae* family (mint) plants.

Appearance: charming perennial herb with a compact and bushy appearance. It typically grows to a height of 6 to 12 inches, with woody stems covered in small, oval-shaped, and aromatic leaves. These leaves are green-gray in color and have a slightly fuzzy texture. During the summer, thyme produces clusters of tiny, delicate flowers in shades of white, pink, or lavender.

Native Habitat: Thyme is native to the Mediterranean region but is widely cultivated and naturalized in various parts of the world. It thrives in sunny and well-drained soil conditions.

Planting Thyme:

Thyme is commonly used in cooking, herbal remedies, and as an ornamental plant in gardens. It's valued for its low-growing habit and attractive small flowers.

- **Soil:** Thyme prefers well-draining soil that is sandy or loamy, with a pH range of 6.0 to 8.0. It can tolerate poor soil conditions, but good drainage is essential for its growth.

- **Light:** Thyme thrives in full sun. It requires at least 6 hours of direct sunlight per day for optimal growth and flavor development.

- **Watering:** Thyme is drought-tolerant once established. Water it deeply but infrequently, allowing the soil to dry out between waterings to prevent root rot.

UNLOCK THE SECRETS OF PLANT MEDICINE AT HOME

- **Fertilizing:** Thyme generally does not require heavy fertilization. However, you can apply a balanced organic fertilizer in early spring or use compost as a top dressing to provide some nutrients.

- **Seasonal adaptability:** Thyme is a perennial herb that is highly adaptable to different climates. It can tolerate both warm and cool temperatures and is generally frost-tolerant.

- **Pruning:** Prune thyme regularly to maintain its shape and encourage bushier growth. Trim back the stems after flowering to promote new growth and prevent the plant from becoming woody.

- **Harvesting:** Harvest thyme leaves as needed throughout the growing season. You can start harvesting once the plant has developed enough foliage. Snip the stems just above a leaf node, and use the fresh or dried leaves in your culinary preparations.

Container Gardening:

When growing thyme in containers, there are a few considerations to keep in mind. First, select a well-draining pot with good drainage holes to prevent waterlogging and root rot. Use a high-quality potting mix that is specifically formulated for container gardening. Thyme prefers full sun, so place the container in a location where it will receive at least 6-8 hours of direct sunlight per day. Regular watering is essential, but be careful not to overwater as thyme prefers slightly drier conditions. Fertilize the plant with a balanced, slow-release fertilizer according to the package instructions. Prune thyme regularly to promote bushier growth and to prevent it from becoming too leggy. Harvest the leaves as needed and remember to bring the container indoors or provide frost protection if temperatures drop below the plant's tolerance.

#36 Valerian – *Valeriana officinalis*

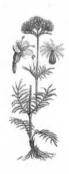

Parts used: roots

Taste: earthy, slightly bitter

Actions: anti-inflammatory, antispasmodic, carminative, sedative,

Preparation and Dosage: Prepare a decoction by simmering 1-2 teaspoons of dried valerian root in a cup of water for 10-15 minutes. Strain and drink before bedtime.

Common uses: Valerian is primarily known for its sedative and calming effects on the nervous system. It is often used as a natural remedy for insomnia, helping to promote restful sleep and alleviate sleep disturbances. Valerian is also valued for its anxiolytic properties, reducing anxiety and promoting a sense of calm. It has antispasmodic effects, making it useful for relieving muscle tension and menstrual cramps. Valerian acts as nervine, supporting and nourishing the nervous system. Additionally, it has carminative properties that help relieve digestive discomfort and promote healthy digestion.

For anxiety relief, take 300-600 mg of valerian extract in capsule form, up to three times per day.

Contraindications: Valerian should not be used during pregnancy or while breastfeeding. It may cause drowsiness, so it is important to avoid activities that require alertness after consuming valerian. Individuals with liver disease should exercise caution when using valerian.

Appearance: Valerian is a perennial herb that grows up to 5 feet in height. It has hollow stems with clusters of small, fragrant flowers that can vary in color from white to pink. The leaves are feathery and divided into smaller leaflets.

Native Habitat: Valerian is native to Europe and parts of Asia, but it is now cultivated in various regions around the world. It prefers moist and well-drained soil conditions and is often found growing near streams or in damp meadows.

Planting Valerian:

Valerian is also a popular plant for gardens in the Midwest. It produces clusters of small, fragrant flowers in the summer, adding beauty to the garden.

- **Soil:** Valerian prefers loamy, well-draining soil that is rich in organic matter. It thrives in moist soil conditions, but it should not be waterlogged.

- **Light:** Valerian prefers full sun to partial shade. It can tolerate some shade but performs best with at least 6 hours of direct sunlight per day.

- **Watering:** Valerian requires regular watering to keep the soil evenly moist. Avoid overwatering, as it can lead to root rot. Monitor the soil moisture and water when the top inch of soil feels dry.

- **Fertilizing:** Valerian does not typically require heavy fertilization. However, you can incorporate compost or well-rotted organic matter into the soil before planting to provide nutrients.

- **Seasonal adaptability:** Valerian is a perennial herb that is adapted to temperate climates. It can tolerate cold temperatures and even frost. It goes dormant during the winter months and regrows in spring.

- **Pruning:** Valerian does not require extensive pruning. However, you can remove spent flowers to encourage continuous blooming and prevent self-seeding.

- **Harvesting:** Valerian roots are typically harvested in the fall of the plant's second or third year. Dig up the roots carefully, clean them, and dry them in a well-ventilated area. The leaves and flowers can also be harvested during the blooming period for medicinal use.

Container Gardening:

Due to its spreading nature, valerian is sometimes grown in containers to control its growth and prevent it from taking over the garden.

#37 Yarrow – *Achillea millefolium*

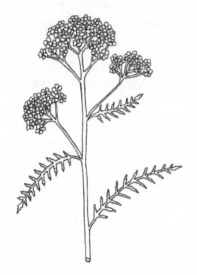

Parts used: aerial parts

Taste: bitter

Actions: diaphoretic, emmenagogue, hypotensive, astringent, anti-inflammatory, diuretic, antimicrobial, alterative, oxytocic

Preparation and Dosage: Place 1 to 2 teaspoons of the dried herb in one cup of boiling water. Strain and take one cup three times daily.

Common uses: Yarrow is a superior diaphoretic for lowering fevers and controlling coughs. It is very suitable for children and the elderly. Please recall this important feature during cold, cough, and flu season. The gentle herb is a steady companion for all in the family.

It also lowers blood pressure by simultaneously stimulating and toning the blood vessels. A simple poultice with Yarrow applied to a wound will stop bleeding.

Yarrow stimulates menstrual flow and help regulate the menstrual cycle.

Contraindications: Please follow the recommended dosage.

Appearance: Herbaceous perennial plant that typically grows to a height of 1 to 3 feet. It has a clumping growth habit with numerous erect stems. The foliage consists of finely divided, feathery leaves that are aromatic when crushed. The flowers of yarrow are small and arranged in flattened clusters called corymbs. They can be white, yellow, pink, or lavender in color and are often visited by pollinators such as bees and butterflies.

Native Habitat: Native to regions across North America, Europe, and Asia. It is commonly found in meadows, fields, grasslands, and open woodlands.

UNLOCK THE SECRETS OF PLANT MEDICINE AT HOME

Planting Yarrow:

With its low maintenance requirements and ability to attract pollinators, yarrow is often included in perennial flower beds, herb gardens, and native plant landscapes in the Midwest.

- **Soil:** Yarrow is adaptable to various soil types but prefers well-draining soil. It can tolerate poor soil conditions and is often found growing in dry or rocky areas.

- **Light:** Yarrow thrives in full sun but can tolerate partial shade. It requires at least 6-8 hours of direct sunlight per day for optimal growth and flowering.

- **Watering:** Yarrow is drought-tolerant once established and does not require frequent watering. It prefers dry to moderately moist soil. Avoid overwatering, as it can lead to root rot.

- **Fertilizing:** Yarrow does not typically require heavy fertilization. It can benefit from a light application of balanced fertilizer in early spring to promote healthy growth.

- **Seasonal adaptability:** Yarrow is a hardy perennial that is adaptable to a wide range of climates. It can tolerate both cold and hot temperatures. It blooms from late spring to summer.

- **Pruning:** Yarrow does not require extensive pruning. Deadheading spent flowers can encourage continuous blooming. Cut back the foliage in late fall or early spring to promote new growth.

- **Harvesting:** Yarrow flowers are typically harvested when they are fully open and vibrant in color. Harvest them in the morning when the essential oils are at their highest concentration. The leaves can also be harvested throughout the growing season for medicinal use.

Container Gardening:

The main difference in growing yarrow in containers compared to outdoor gardening is the limited space and restricted root growth. In containers, yarrow has a more confined root system, which can affect its overall size and spread. Additionally, container-grown yarrow may require more frequent watering as the soil in containers tends to dry out faster. Adequate drainage becomes crucial in container gardening to prevent waterlogging and root rot. Some yarrow varieties may also require staking or support in containers to prevent them from flopping over. Overall, container gardening offers the advantage of portability and control over soil quality and moisture levels, but it requires closer monitoring and adjustment of growing conditions compared to outdoor gardening.

#38 Yellow Dock – *Rumex crispus*

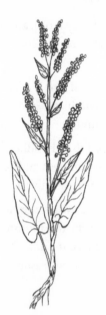

Parts Used: root

Temperature: cooling

Actions: alterative, cholagogue, blood tonic, astringent

Preparation and Dosage: Use the Standard Decoction of the roots to make the tea. Use one teaspoon of the dried root per cup of boiling water.

Contraindications: Use the Yellow Curly Dock roots, not the leaves, on this variety.

Common uses: Yellow Dock root is a beneficial herb for imbalances resulting from excessive liver and colon heat. It clears liver congestion and is a mild purgative for the large intestine. Indeed, it does have a laxative effect, but its star quality rests in treating anemia.

Appearance: Perennial herb that belongs to the buckwheat family. It typically grows to a height of 2 to 4 feet and has a robust and erect stem. The leaves are large, elongated, and lance-shaped with prominent veins. They have a slightly wrinkled or wavy texture and can range in color from deep green to reddish-brown. Yellow Dock produces small, greenish-yellow flowers in elongated clusters that rise above the foliage. The plant's root system consists of a long taproot.

Native Habitat: Native to Europe and western Asia. It has naturalized in various regions around the world, including North America, where it is often considered an invasive weed. Yellow Dock thrives in disturbed areas, such as fields, roadsides, and waste areas.

Planting in Gardens and Containers:

Yellow Dock are typically not intentionally planted in gardens or pots, as they are considered weeds by many gardeners. But the chances are high you will find them in your garden or public area.

6   Tools and techniques for Making Your Own Herbal Medicine

6.1   Supplies Needed for Preparing Herbal Formulas

Stocking your supplies to make remedies before you start collecting herbs is important. You will feel unprepared if you end up with an herb without the objects necessary for preparation.

Here is a list of what you need:

- Cheesecloth to strain your remedies — One main benefit of cheesecloth is that you can squeeze it when you strain it to remove the core of the botanical extracts. Note: in a pinch, you can also use a coffee filter.

- Mortar and pestle for making spice blends.

- An assortment of funnels.

- Clean, sanitized jars (2oz, 4oz, 8oz, and 16oz) A variety of jars means that no matter what amount of an herb you procure, you are ready to store it properly.

- A double boiler to condense some of your formulas and create salves. if you don't have one at home then just put a bowl in a cooking pot.

- Parchment paper or clean paper bags to dry your herbs on

- String to tie your herbs and hang them to dry.

- Cotton or flannel cloths (a dishtowel works well) to cut up and use for poultices and compresses.

- A few ounces of beeswax to make salves.

- At least 12 ounces of olive oil to make oil extractions and salves.

- Two-ounce dropper bottles (brown or blue) to make your first tincture. Order a dozen to start. A two-ounce bottle will yield three doses of 1 inch, or one dropper full, for about twenty-five days.

- Optional: you can order tea bags online or you can simply strain your loose tea.

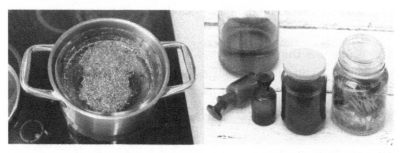

Picture left: Self-made 'double boiler' with a bowl in a cooking pot. Right: jars for storing herbs and herbal remedies. Remember to store them in a dark, cool place.

6.2 How to Harness the Power of Herbs

Many people are terrified at the thought of making their own medicine. This common fear can be alleviated by simply understanding what is involved in the process and getting to know the qualities of the plants themselves. You will be very encouraged to learn that, overall, the risks of herbal medicine making are quite low. With all due respect, most master herbalists, herbal teachers, and a growing number of physicians are well aware of the fact that fewer lives have been harmed by herbs than by the consequences of relying exclusively on pharmaceutical prescriptions.

You already add natural medicinal spices to your food, you already make tea, and you may have followed your grandmother's advice about taking a natural remedy. Plus, just picking up this book shows you are eager to learn about natural healing. You are already qualified! Rest assured in the competence of our ancient teachers. Herbalism is both an art and a science, finely tuned over thousands of years.

We have to bear in mind that formulation techniques used today differ in some ways from traditional preparations. In previous sections, we have seen how they used teas, baths, and chewing the herb directly (e.g. as a tea). Other common uses included poultices, compresses, and salves.

Unless one uses the herb directly, herbs require a liquid menstruum, or medium, to dissolve their active ingredients so the body can absorb them. One extracts the primary medicinal herbal components into the so-called 'menstruum' to different potency levels that harness the power of the herb.

Here are the main ones:

1. Water — is used for teas, steaming and baths, compresses, poultices, and oral swishes.

2. Water as a menstruum is gentle and easily absorbed. Hot water breaks down herbal components.

3. Alcohol — for instance vodka, or another type of liquor used for tinctures kept in dropper bottles is a superior menstruum. Alcohol is advantageous because it breaks down the oils in herbs like tannins that contain valuable healing properties.

4. Vinegar — used in the same way as alcohol to extract herbal properties to make tonics, administered by teaspoon. Vinegar is a helpful medium because its extraction power is just a bit below alcohol but it contains other properties that optimize digestion.

5. Honey — is a good menstruum for children's formulas like syrups, administered by teaspoon.

6. Glycerin — is a good menstruum for children's formulas or for people who cannot tolerate alcohol tinctures, administered by teaspoon. Glycerin provides an alternative to honey, is tolerated by those who cannot have alcohol and is inexpensive.

UNLOCK THE SECRETS OF PLANT MEDICINE AT HOME

7. Oil — is used to extract herbal properties to make massage oils and salves.

8. Oil is advantageous because it allows people to make their own topical applications.

6.3 Water-Based Remedies: Infusions, Decoctions, Herbal Steaming, Herbal Baths, Foot Soaks, Oral Swishes, Compresses, Poultices

Infusions

Infusions are teas made with leaves and flowers. If you have made a delicious cup of tea at any point in your life, you are perfectly qualified to create infusions. The only difference is understanding how to administer the correct medicinal dose.

The medicinal dosage of tea for a chronic condition is three cups a day. However, it is very tedious to make a cup at a time. Make three quarts of tea at time if you are taking a remedy for more than a week. Take your daily dose of three cups of your preferred tea and store the other two quarts in the refrigerator.

Making tea in advance is practical. If you are sick, you don't want to get in and out of bed all of the time and disturb your sleep, just to make tea.

Of all the remedies, teas are the easiest to make:

1. Boil your water, and put your herbs in a small pot for infusion.

2. Traditionally, one teaspoon of dried herb, or one tablespoon of chopped fresh herbs is required per cup of water. A storebought tea bag typically contains a teaspoon of a dried substance.

3. Cover your herbs with the boiled water and steep for 15 minutes. Hot water is your menstruum. It breaks down the components of an herb. Remember, heat creates movement so you are making it possible for your herbs to move throughout your body and complete their actions.

4. Strain and store in a glass jar.

5. Infusions are bursting with life and therefore attract microorganisms! Make sure to discard your tea after storing it if it tastes fermented or smells spoiled.

Tea works with the body in a unique way. Our bodies are made of roughly 80% water. An herbal tea infusion is a remedy that balances the water content in your body. The medicinal tea ingredients carried in water flush unwanted bacteria and toxins from various systems.

If you want, you can order muslin or paper tea bags to make your own tea bags.

Decoctions

Decoctions are similar to infusions, but they are required for a more sensitive medium like a bark, seed or a root. The proportions are the same, either 1 teaspoon of dried root, seed, or bark, or 1 tablespoon of fresh root, seed or bark per cup of water. Mint is a leaf so you will infuse it, while Ginger is a root, so you will decoct that.

1. Slowly simmer the decoction for twenty minutes. Add a little water at the end to make up for the evaporation.

2. Strain and store in a glass jar.

3. Teas made with barks or roots tend to last up to a week when refrigerated. Make one to three quarts at a time.

Herbal Steams/Epsom Salts Baths/Foot Soaks

Herbal steams with essential oils, herbal baths and herb foot soaks with hot water are important methods for clearing stagnation, reducing infection, for nourishment, and simple restoration.

Herbal Steaming

If an herb is aromatic, like mint leaves, roses or lemon balm you can make an infusion in a small pot and create a tent over your head with a towel to breathe in the aroma. Different herbs like mint for instance clear the nasal passages and also are sedative.

1. Chop 1 tablespoon of fresh leaves or roots and place them in 1 quart of boiling water.

2. Make a tent over your head with a hand towel and put your face at least a foot above the steam. You do not want to burn your skin.

3. Inhale until the smell fades.

4. Dry your face off and cover up to prevent any exposure from the cold. Rest if needed.

5. Repeat this three to five times per day depending on the condition. If it is chronic three times is fine. If it is acute, five times may be required.

Herbal Baths

Soaking in an herbal bath is basically like drinking an enormous cup of tea (safely of course). Your skin is the largest organ in your body; it absorbs nutrients and also expels toxins through its pores. Baths are a time-tested form of healing.

For instance, to stop a child's diarrhea place the child in a small tub of blackberry leaf infused water. Absorbing the water through their skin in a hot tub is relaxing. It avoids the issue of trying to give a bitter tea to a child to ingest.

Prepare a bath using the following steps:

For a fresh herbal bath:

1. Take two cups of a chopped herb tied up in cheesecloth. Place this in 4 cups of boiling water, for leaves, infuse for 15 minutes, for roots, seeds and bark decoct for 20 minutes.

2. Cool and strain your tea.

3. Run your bath water.

4. Put the tea in your bath. For a bath using essential oils:
   - o Run a hot bath and put 15–20 drops of essential oil in the bath.
   - o Swish it around with your hand to disperse it before you get in the bathtub.
   - o Stay in the bath for at least fifteen minutes so that your skin can absorb the oils.

Don't use mint oil in the bathtub! It is too cooling and does not break down as well in the hot water so ironically, it can also burn the skin.

Foot Soaks

A foot soak works in the same way as a bath and is tolerated more easily by those who cannot get into the bathtub.

1. Use ½ cup of chopped herbs.

2. Tie them in a square of cheesecloth.

3. Heat three-quart of water.

4. Find a suitable chair for the person to sit and place a towel on the floor in front of the chair.

5. Put the foot tub on the towel and fill it with hot water.

6. Place the three cups of herbal water that you have either infused or decocted into the tub.

7. A person can sit and relax here for up to a half-hour absorbing the herbal benefits.

8. Dry the feet and put on a pair of cotton socks to let the skin breathe.

9. Once or twice a day for a chronic condition should be enough.

Oral Swishes

Oral swishes are an excellent form of preventative dental care and maintenance. They can also help reduce canker sores, toothaches or any other sore in the mouth.

An **oral swish** occurs when you use a tincture or strong tea and continually swish it in your mouth to decrease inflammation and infection. Maybe you have already done this with simple warm salt water, for instance, to reduce an abscess. You will find a recipe for a Sage oral swish in this book.

1. Take 1" or tincture or 1 tablespoon of strong tea into the oral cavity. Tea or tincture will vary depending on the ailment you wish to treat.

2. Swish the liquid in the oral cavity but do not swallow it. Let it touch the inner surfaces of the mouth so it is absorbed.

3. After ten minutes, spit it out in the garbage.

Let the liquid soak into the oral tissues and follow up by drinking a glass of water after another ten minutes or so.

Compresses

Making a compress is a lot like making a cup of tea. However, you must have a square cotton or flannel cloth on hand for topical application.

1. Make a cup of tea with one cup of boiling water and 1 teaspoon of the chosen herb (for example, Ginger to reduce inflammation).

2. Fold a flannel or cotton cloth into a square.

3. Strain the tea and pour it into a bowl.

4. When it has cooled down so you can touch it, soak the cloth in it. Make sure that it is still warm.

5. Ring out the cloth and apply to the affected area for twenty minutes. You can repeat this process three times a day, or repeatedly in acute cases of inflammation.

Poultices

A poultice is usually made from an herbal paste, a chopped and cooked herb, or in an emergency a quickly macerated herb. It is spread on an injury, ache or wound. You will hold this paste in place with a cloth. A poultice can pull infections and toxins from an affected area or heal a wound.

1. Prepare a half cup of herbs by the infusion or decoction method. Another example is baking soda in water to make a paste.

2. Strain and place on the affected area.

3. Cover with a flannel or cotton cloth and hold for twenty minutes. You can tie a band around the cloth to hold it in place.

4. Dry the area but do not scrape it. Let the herbal residue continue to soak in.

5. Reapply as needed depending on the condition.

6.4   Tinctures

Tinctures

Tinctures are made with alcohol, vinegar, honey, and glycerin. Tinctures concentrate the active components of the herbs through the process of extraction. **Extraction is the heart of formulating herbal remedies.** Concentrated extractions release the active components of herbs to enable healing.

Alcohol is uniquely effective at extracting the components of an herb, releasing them into the menstruum. For those who cannot tolerate alcohol, like children, some tinctures in this book will be made with vinegar, honey, or glycerin.

This book teaches the simpling method and only gives a recipe for one more complex antiviral formula. An alcohol tincture is the easiest way to make a remedy, besides making tea.

The simpling method is a traditional approach to herbal medicine that involves using a single herb at a time for medicinal purposes. It emphasizes the use of whole herbs in their natural form, such as leaves, flowers, or roots, rather than isolated compounds or extracts. The method focuses on simplicity and the direct use of herbs in various preparations, such as teas, infusions, poultices, or herbal baths.

Using the simpling method, you will cover your herbs in a glass jar with the menstruum you are using. Generally, it ends up balancing a 50% to 50% ratio, herb/menstruum. If your herbs soak up the menstruum, simply add more menstruum, for example alcohol, to the top until it covers the herb. Do not add water to your tinctures or they will attract mold.

The simpling method has been practiced for thousands of years. A huge benefit is that if you find a remedy and make a batch of it, for less than fifty dollars a batch you will have enough remedy for six months at the chronic dose level.

People certainly have their preferences for the type of alcohol used. Mainly, it needs to be at least 60 proof in order to break down the herbs (primarily the oils, terpenes in them). Plain vodka is generally recommended, especially if you are just starting out. It is easy to work with, effective and has little taste.

1. Start with a clean jar. If your jars and lids are not clean, your medicine might acquire fungus or bacteria.

2. Put your herbs in the bottom and add your menstruum, in this case, alcohol over the herbs.

3. Close the jar and let this sit in a dark place, with a neutral temperature, for twenty-one days. (The twenty-one-day waiting period is a traditional ancient practice.)

4. After twenty-one days, line a strainer with cheesecloth and strain your tincture into a bowl.

5. Gather the edges of the cheesecloth and twist them until you squeeze out the very last drop of your medicine. Those last drops contain the highest concentration of ingredients from your herbs.

6. Use a funnel or a vessel with a spout to pour your herbal liquid into a glass jar for storage.

7. Cap and store in a cool dark place. The mixture will store for several years or more.

Alcohol tinctures can be stored for the longest period of time. Consequently, they are convenient and cost-effective.

6.5   Using Vinegar, Honey or Glycerin

Vinegar

Vinegar contains acetic acid and is a solvent and preservative like alcohol, only not quite as strong. You would follow the same simpling procedure using vinegar for tonic preparations.

The benefit of using vinegar is that it is non-toxic and tolerated by almost everyone. People who cannot drink alcohol can consume vinegar. It has excellent nutritional benefits; it restores your microbiome (the lining of your gut) and rejuvenates the health of the digestive tract. Vinegar has a slightly laxative effect.

Glycerin

Glycerin is used for children and in some cases for adults who cannot handle alcohol. It does not break down oils and resins as well as alcohol or vinegar. The tincturing process is different from the simpling method.

1. Dilute the glycerin with water by half 50% to 50%.

2. Cover your herbs with the diluted glycerin and strain after two to three weeks.

3. Store your syrup in a clean glass jar.

Honey

Honey as a menstruum is in a category alone. Sometimes referred to as an 'elixir', it is a powerful menstruum. It is a great way to deliver medicine to children, and those resistant to herbal preparations. There are two main ways to prepare medicine using honey.

1. You can soak certain herbs in honey by covering them with honey and letting them sit in a cool dark place for three weeks or longer. The honey, after a couple of weeks will break the herbal components down and extract them. For instance, you could make Ginger, Garlic or Rose elixir in this manner.

Or use the second method:

2. Infuse or decoct your herbs in a pot on the stove, cool, strain, and add the honey afterward. An example of this method is Elderberry syrup, discussed in the recipe section.

6.6 Taking Herbal Powders

Bake Herbal Pills and Alternative Ways of Consumption

Making your own herbal pills is a time-consuming process. Purchasing pills is an option. Better yet, you can take the powder in a medium such as:

- Yogurt
- Pudding
- Oatmeal
- Juice

The standard dosage of herbal powders is 500mg three times daily. This varies, however, depending on the herbal substance.

500mg equals ½ teaspoon in general

One option is to place ½ teaspoon of herbal powder in a small cup, mix it with one of the choices listed above and swallow. You would do this three times daily for a chronic condition.

Adjust the child's dose as needed. Alternatively, look at the herbal cookie recipe in Chapter 8.3 'Immunity'. It provides a more interesting way for your family to take medicine. You can use the cookies preventatively to boost the immune system or when a child gets sick, if they can swallow them, as a 'treat'. Another tasty alternative is lozenges.

Herbal Powder in Lozenges as Herbal Medicine

You will be surprised how simple it is to prepare your own throat lozenges.

1. Prepare one ounce of Tragacanth (a natural gum you can order online) by melting it in 1 pint of boiling water.
2. After melting, soak the mixture for twenty-four hours.
3. The following day, beat the mixture to make it smooth.
4. Strain it through two layers of cheesecloth to make a gummy liquid.
5. Add 1 tablespoon of brown sugar.
6. Add 2 tablespoons or more of the herbal powder you choose.
7. Put cornflour on a surface to roll out the paste.
8. Roll out the paste covering it with the cornflour.
9. Let it cool and then cut it into squares.
10. Store the lozenges in a tin or glass container.

Take the lozenges as needed depending on the amount of herbal powder in each lozenge.

6.7 Oils and Salves

Oil Infusions (Oleolites)

When a plant is extracted in oil it is called an oleolite. Usually, an oleolite will alleviate skin issues, including inflammation. It is always a good idea to keep an oil extraction handy for making your salves, for use as massage oil, or for aches and pains. If you use just the right ingredients, for instance roses, your oil extraction serves as a beauty product as well.

1. In a quart sized jar place 1 cup of your dried herb, or two cups of a fresh herb.

2. Cover the herb completely with whatever oil you choose (olive, almond, avocado, and apricot are good choices).

3. Cover the jar with a lid.

4. Store in a cool, dark place for thirty to forty days. It takes a long time for oil extractions to finish. Oil is a very dense menstruum.

5. Shake the jar a couple of times a week to mix your ingredients.

6. After the extraction is finished, strain the oil into a strainer lined with cheesecloth that sits over a bowl.

7. After the oil drips through the cloth, gather the edges of the cloth and twist and squeeze all of the oil out into the bowl.

8. Pour the finished extraction into a glass jar.

9. Store in a cool, dark place. Oleolites have a fair degree of shelf stability and will last for a couple of years when stored properly.

Salves

Salves are applied topically only. Many people turn to salves because if they contain anti-inflammatory herbs, they are an effective alternative to using NSAIDs[1] For salves, the oil extractions you make will be your menstruum.

Here is the general recipe for a salve:

1. Warm 1 cup of herbal extracted oil you have prepared in a double boiler.

2. Add ¼ cup of beeswax and stir until melted.

---

1   Non-steroidal anti-inflammatory drugs (NSAIDs) are medicines that are widely used to relieve pain, reduce inflammation including acetaminophen and ibuprofen.

3. Pour into small jars or metal tins. Cap and store in a cool, dark place.

6.8 Aromatherapy

Aromatherapy began with the practice of smelling the plant itself. Just smelling a rose or rosemary bush has a healing effect. Aromatherapy involves using a very concentrated essence of the plants.

It is not an oleation (the practice of applying or ingesting oils or oily substances as part of therapeutic treatments). An aromatic essential oil is much more concentrated. It takes thirty to fifty roses to produce one drop of rose essential oil! Two hundred and fifty pounds of lavender produces one pound of lavender essential oils. The underlying principle of aromatherapy is "less is more". Aromatherapy is a vast science in and of itself and it is not possible to go into depth in this book.

With just a few drops, a person can achieve powerful results, particularly when it comes to mood alteration and alleviating skin issues. European chemists refined the practice of aromatherapy through steam distillation although simple oil extractions have been used for hundreds of years.

Essential oils heal in two main ways:

1. The aroma itself triggers the olfactory sense and acts on specific neurochemicals to achieve desired results.

2. The oils, when they contact tissue surfaces are absorbed, bind to fat cells, and then act on specific neurotransmitters.

3. Memories of smells are powerful. When a memory of an essential oil smell combines with the effect it has on the body a person retains an impression of its ability to heal. For instance, if you use lavender oil before sleeping and it actually helps you fall asleep, the next time a person smells lavender oil they are likely to react.

Essential oils are very convenient, save time and are cost-effective. Just by keeping the following short list on hand, you can address multiple

UNLOCK THE SECRETS OF PLANT MEDICINE AT HOME

conditions. Starting an apothecary by purchasing a few essential oils is an easy way for you to start creating your home apothecary.

Please note: One cannot put essential oils directly on the skin. You have to dissolve them first in a substance.

Dissolve essentials oils in:

1. Hot water

   o   As a general rule, put three to five drops in a small pot for steaming. For a child, one drop will be enough.

   o   Twenty drops in a bathtub — remember to put the drops in the bath and swish them around thoroughly.

2. A carrier lotion or oil

   o   3 drops per half teaspoon of oil is a general rule.

Steaming with Essential Oils

You can keep a ready supply of essential oils on hand for steaming if fresh herbs are not available.

There are 1,000 drops of essential oil in a 1-ounce vial. That is a compact form of healing and you can take these vials with you when you travel!

For steaming a good rule of thumb to follow is to use one drop for every 30 pounds you carry. If you weigh a hundred and thirty pounds, you will need about four drops.

When building your apothecary, keep one to two ounces of the following on hand:

- Peppermint — Please read the Materia Medica on this herb. Using the essential oil is optional in cases where a person does not want to ingest peppermint. Mint is far too potent to use on the skin. Primarily you can steam with three drops of the oil under a steam tent as needed to open the sinus cavities. Mint is a very strong essential oil.

- Tea Tree — is an excellent antibacterial oil that can be used on the skin (five drops to ½ teaspoon of carrier oil) for all types of bug bites, stings, and minor infections. Adjust the dose for children. One or two drops per ½ teaspoon is plenty.

- Lavender — is a superior remedy for anxiety, and a sleep aid (five drops for ½ teaspoon of carrier oil) to heal minor wounds, burns, and insect bites. Apply to the back of the neck. Adjust the dose for children. One drop per ½ teaspoon is generally plenty for a child over the age of three or four depending on how much they weigh.

- Eucalyptus — is a great remedy for steaming in case of cold, cough, or flu. It is an expectorant. Four drops for an adult in a small pot of steaming water is enough. This oil is OK for older children but probably too strong for younger children unless it is used in a diffuser specifically designed to permeate a room with an essence.

7   Guidelines for Using Remedies

Let's turn to the details of constructing your daily apothecary, stocking required herbs, and combining various remedies for everyday use.

To prepare your home apothecary, familiarize yourself with the following principles to store your remedies and make them readily available:

1. Dosages for adults and children
2. The amount of herbs to keep on hand for the most basic situations
3. How to sequence the stages of a condition to know what herb to take at which stage

Everyone has the gift to heal. However, it requires skill and experience to treat yourself. Look carefully under the conditions in these guidelines to see what applies to the illness you are dealing with. The table on Chapter 9 gives an overview of the herbs to use for different issues that you wish to address.

Notice the stages of illness and the possibilities of healing at each stage using different remedies. Be aware of conditions that may become too advanced for you to treat on your own. Seek help when needed from a qualified holistic practitioner.

Please note: You can improve the taste of most teas with just a couple of pinches of either lemon zest, orange zest, or powdered mint. Honey is always an option.

Please review the following chapter regarding dosage carefully. You will have more clarity about the quantity of herbs needed for storage and, even more importantly, for consumption. Remember that you can usually buy common herbs by the ounce in your local health food store or co-op. Otherwise, you may harvest or grow them or purchase them in bulk online.

7.1   Learning About Herbal Dosages

Many of the herbs you gather will be mild. Therefore, the dosage of mild herbs may be higher, and the intake duration lengthened to make a difference in a long-term chronic condition. It is worth noting: master herbalists point out that **most mistakes made when taking herbs occur due to taking the wrong dosage.** Generally, the dose taken is too low, and so the person assumes that an herb is ineffective.

Remember that:

1. The standard herbal tea dose for a chronic condition is three cups a day.

2. The usual dose of an alcohol-based tincture is 1" or one dropper full three times daily.

3. The standard dosage of an herbal pill for chronic conditions is 500 mg to 1000 mg three times daily.

4. The usual dose of syrup is one teaspoon three times daily.

Commonly, people assume that they only need a pinch of herbs to make a difference, almost like the amount of spice you use to add flavor to a dish. But no, the human body is more complex than cooking a meal. This complexity must be considered even as a beginner when administering an herb. Please take the dosage instructions in this book seriously. Ask yourself the following questions if an herb does not work for you:

1. Would you be willing to take a larger dose if your herb is mild?

2. Do you need to have more patience with your healing process and wait for the herb to take effect?

3. Do you eat processed foods, foods out of season, or foods from other climates that slow your healing process down?

4. Is your healing process affected by any other lifestyle factors?

5. Do you need to see a practitioner for guidance? Encourage yourself to get the support you need.

Overall, remember that emphasizing elements such as slowing down, nurturing family and community connections, immersing in nature, reevaluating priorities, and seeking support are equally crucial alongside herbal remedies. These aspects play a vital role in fostering holistic well-being, making them essential in our daily lives.

Simple conversion of mass units

Bulk herbs are generally sold by the ounce. Most herbal companies require a minimum purchase of 4 ounces. Conversions from ounces to tablespoons and teaspoons follow.

Common Measurement Conversions for Herbal Substances

1 ounce = 2 tablespoons and 6 teaspoons

2 ounces = 4 tablespoons and 12 teaspoons

4 ounces = 8 tablespoons and 24 teaspoons

7.2 Self-Monitoring and when to Seek Medical Support

Learn the baselines first. Check-in with yourself daily. Do you notice any changes? Three times daily means morning, afternoon, and evening. Carry your tincture, tea, pills, or syrup in your purse or backpack so that you will not miss a dose when you leave the house.

Last but not least — drink plenty of water! Herbs act on particular systems and often release toxins from them. Astringent herbs literally squeeze liquid from the cells to release excesses and allow room for cells to renew. It takes extra water to facilitate all of the jobs that herbs perform.

1. Do you feel dehydrated after taking your herbs?
2. Do you feel a headache after taking your herb?
3. Do you feel nausea after taking your herb?

If any of these feelings apply to you, try drinking more water. If that does not help, call a practitioner.

7.3   Remedies fo Kids

If not indicated differently, kids can take the same remedies as adults but with different dosages. To determine the right dosage for children, let's look at Cowling's rule. It is a formula to calculate a dose of herbs for children. Getting children to taste medicine is not always easy. You have to be creative. Sometimes children (or adults for that matter) take medicine more easily in yogurt, applesauce, or pudding. Do whatever works for the individual.

Cowling's Rule is the year of the child's next birthday divided by 24. So if your child turns four next year and you divide four by 24 you will administer 1/6 of the adult dosage.[2]

Children often like tea. It is comforting and warm and especially if you put a little honey in it, they usually drink it. An adult tea dosage is one cup. For a child give the following amount of tea:

1. Children 1 year or less — two teaspoons
2. Children 2 to 4 years — three teaspoons
3. Children 4 to 7 years — 1 tablespoon
4. Children 7 to 11 years — 2 tablespoons

---

2   Gladstar, Rosemary, "Art and Science of Herbalism", Chapter 4, p.7

8 Collection of Herbal Remedies Suiting your Needs

8.1 Remedies with Various Uses

Remember, that the effectiveness of herbal remedies can vary from person to person, and it may depend on individual responses and the specific circumstances of an ailment. Each herb may have slightly different effects and potency, so it's essential to try them individually to see which one works best for you.

This book focuses on remedies that represent a choice of the most common and widely accepted uses of each herb. While there are many uses for each herb, certain remedies are repeatedly mentioned for specific ailments. To avoid redundancy in manufacturing instructions, this chapter compiles those remedies. They will be marked with (**) so you know that the detailed description is available in this chapter.

For each recommended remedy that is not mentioned in this chapter, you will find either an immediate manufacturing description in the text or you need to go back to Chapter 6, where you can learn how to manufacture it using a specific menstruum.

The remedies mentioned severally in this book are:

Antiviral Tincture (Boneset/ Butterfly Weed Root/ Meadowsweet/ Lemon Balm/ Ginseng)

This recipe is a little more complex than a simpling recipe using one herb, but the same principle applies. You will combine the herbs and then cover them completely with alcohol.

Combine:

- ounces Boneset (reduce fever, body ache, and coughing)
- ounces Butterfly Weed Root (expectorant, reduces fever, dispels toxins)
- 2 ounces Meadowsweet (anti-inflammatory and pain-relieving)
- 2 ounces Lemon Balm (calming and Relaxing, antiviral, antioxidant)
- 2 ounces Ginseng (immunostimulant, increases stamina)

Place ingredients in a glass jar. Cover with alcohol and let sit in a cool dark place for 21 days—strain and store in a glass jar. You can also put your tincture into 2-ounce dropper bottles.

If you get the flu, which is an acute condition, at the onset of symptoms, you will need to begin taking this tincture 1" at least every four hours. As symptoms persist or even increase, take this tincture 1" every three hours. Decrease the dose gradually as symptoms decrease.

Keep taking the chronic dose three times daily for a week even after symptoms subside. Viruses have a way of embedding themselves deep inside the tissues. Viruses like to hide. Taking this tincture for an additional week ensures that the deeper levels of the illness subside.

Arnica Oil Extraction

1. In a quart-sized jar, place 1 cup of your dried herb or two cups of a fresh herb.
2. Cover the herb entirely with whatever oil you choose (olive, almond, avocado, and apricot are good choices)
3. Cover the jar with a lid.
4. Store in a cool, dark place for thirty to forty days. It takes a long time for oil extractions to complete.
5. Shake the jar a couple of times a week to mix your ingredients.
6. After the extraction is finished, pour the oil into a strainer lined with cheesecloth that sits over a bowl.

7. After the oil drips through the cloth, gather the edges of the cloth. Twist and squeeze all of the oil into the bowl, utilizing the last drop of your extraction.

8. Pour the finished extraction into a glass jar.

9. Store in a cool, dark place. Oleolites have a fair degree of shelf stability and will last for a couple of years when stored properly.

Chamomile Tea

1. Boil one quart of water.

2. Add 1 heaping tablespoon of dried chamomile.

3. Infuse the herbs for 15 minutes.

4. Strain them into a clean glass vessel

5. Drink three cups, morning, afternoon, and evening. Most teas store for three to four days.

Calendula/ Lavender/ St. John's Wort -Infused Oil

You will need 4 oz of dried calendula / lavender/ St. John's Wort flowers to make the infused oil.

1. Prepare the calendula/ lavender/ St. John's Wort -infused oil by filling a glass jar with the dried calendula/ lavender flowers and covering them with the carrier oil.

2. Let the mixture sit in a sunny spot for about 4-6 weeks, shaking it occasionally.

3. Strain the oil and use it topically to soothe skin inflammation and irritations.

After the infusion period, strain the oil and store it in a dark, airtight container.

Elderberry Syrup

Combine:

- One cup of dried elderberries
- One tablespoon grated ginger Three whole cloves
- One cinnamon stick
- 1/2 teaspoon of orange zest Three cups of boiling water
- ¾ cup of honey

In a medium-sized saucepan, heat the water until it boils. Add the elderberries and turn the heat down to simmer. Add the ginger, cloves, cinnamon stick, and orange zest. Continue to simmer and reduce the syrup by half.

Strain into a bowl or measuring cup.

(Discard the berries or boil them again in three cups of water to make tea!)

Add the honey at the end and stir well.

Put the mixture into a glass jar and label it. Elderberry syrup lasts up to eight weeks in the refrigerator.

Take one teaspoon every three hours in case of flu. Take one teaspoon three times a day for a cold or cough.

St. John's Wort

1. Harvest fresh St. John's Wort flowers and leaves.
2. Dry the plant material in a well-ventilated area away from direct sunlight until they are completely dry.
3. Grind the dried plant material into a fine powder using a mortar and pestle or a grinder.
4. Mix the powdered St. John's Wort with a carrier oil of your choice, such as olive oil or coconut oil, to create a soothing and healing herbal oil.

5. Allow the mixture to infuse for 4-6 weeks in a sealed glass jar, shaking it gently daily to ensure proper infusion.

6. After the infusion period, strain the oil through a fine mesh strainer or cheesecloth to remove the plant material.

7. Your St. John's Wort oil is now ready for use. Apply it topically to wounds, bruises, ulcers, cuts, burns, or hemorrhoids to promote healing and alleviate discomfort.

8.2   Your Basic Herbal First Aid Kit

This chapter contains remedies you can store in your apothecary table to face acute situations described below. Test them to find out which ones work best for treating yourself, members of your family or other people you want to treat. Additional remedies for the same conditions are given in later chapters.

Remember, that to avoid redundancy in manufacturing instructions, remedies severally recurring are marked with (**) and are described in chapter 8.1.

Pain and Inflammation

- **Arnica Oil (**)**

    Keep 4oz of Arnica aerial parts and 4 oz olive oil on hand.

    Use for acute or sudden pain, bruises, swelling, and inflammation, for instance from an injury or surgery. Use **Arnica Oil** every three to four hours. Not for cuts or on skin that is not intact. You will need 4 oz of Arnica aerial parts to create the Oil.

- **Calendula-Infused Oil**

    For skin inflammation and irritations and skin health (**)

    Keep 4 oz of dried calendula flowers and 8 oz of carrier oil (such as olive oil or coconut oil) on hand.

    Apply the calendula-infused oil topically to promote skin health.

- **Comfrey Leaf Poultice**

  Blend half a dozen fresh leaves in a blender and mix them with water to create a paste. Optionally, you can add flour or clay to the mixture to improve its consistency. Spread the paste on a cloth in the size of the affected area and put it on the skin, closed wounds, muscles, and joints. You can put the paste in a zip log bag and store it in the freezer to use when needed.

- **Comfrey Root Powder** is mixed with water to form a paste and applied to the affected areas of the skin.

  To prepare the root powder, the freshly harvested root is sliced, quickly dried on a heater or preferably in a dehydrator at a maximum temperature of 95 °F, and then ground into a powder.

  For bruises, sprains, strains, tendonitis, as well as muscle and bone injuries and arthritis (chronic pain).

- **Oregano Essential Oil for Topical Use:**

  This remedy can be handy for quick first aid situations.

  Keep a small bottle of oregano essential oil on hand. Apply a few drops of the oil directly to minor cuts and wounds to help prevent infection and promote healing. Remember to dilute the essential oil with a carrier oil (such as coconut oil) if you have sensitive skin.

- **St. John's Wort (**)**

  Keep 4 oz of St. John's Wort flowers and 8 oz of carrier oil (such as olive oil) on hand.

  Apply topically.

Burns and Cuts

Minor burns and cuts need immediate attention.

- **Plantain Leaf Poultice**

  For burns or cuts.

  Keep 6 oz of cut leaves on hand.

- **Lavender-Infused Oil or Balm**

  For soothing minor cuts and burns (**)

  Keep 4 oz of dried lavender flowers and 8 oz of carrier oil (such as olive or coconut oil) on hand.

- **St. John's Wort (**)**

  Topical treatment of wounds, bruises, ulcers, cuts, burns, hemorrhoids.

Stop Bleeding

If you get a cut in the kitchen or while doing gardening, making a **Yarrow** poultice will stop the bleeding. After the bleeding has stopped, ultimately, you can make a **Plantain** poultice to heal the skin.

- **Yarrow Leaf Poultice**

  Keep 4oz of yarrow leaves on hand.

  Subdues fever or makes a poultice to stop bleeding.

Toothache

- **Sage leaf tea**

  Keep 4 oz — 8 oz Sage leaf on hand.

  It is beneficial to have a decent amount of Sage on hand. One of them is to stop a toothache. Make a cup of Sage tea. Keep it in a jar in the refrigerator and swish with a tablespoon of the tea in your mouth four times daily.

- **Sage Oral Swish**

  For a toothache or teeth whitening

  1. Make a cup of Sage tea using the standard dosage method of 1 teaspoon of dried herb to one cup of boiling water.

  2. Let the tea steep for 15 minutes.

  3. Strain the tea.

4. Swish one tablespoon of the tea in your mouth for 15 minutes. You can also hold the tea with your mouth over the affected tooth for several seconds. Then continue to swish.

5. Spit the tea out.

6. Save the remainder of the tea in a glass jar in the refrigerator.

7. Repeat the process until you feel the pain subside.

Dental pain may be a sign that further care is required. Please see the following for a more comprehensive perspective on holistic dental care.[3]

Fever

- Yarrow leaf tea Keep 4 oz on hand.

Subdues fever or stops bleeding when you apply a poultice.

Cold or Sinus Infection

- **Peppermint Essential Oil Steam**

Keep a 1 oz bottle on hand for steaming.

- **Yarrow Tea**

For fever, cold, and cough

Yarrow tea will reduce fever, cold, or cough. Yarrow is packed with minerals!

How it's done:

1. Boil one quart of water.

2. Add three teaspoons of dried Yarrow leaves.

3. Infuse for 15 minutes.

4. Strain into a clean glass vessel.

5. Drink three cups, morning, afternoon, and evening. Adjust the dose for children.

Most teas store for three to four days.

---

3   Alexander, Leslie M., PhD, RH (AHG) and Linda A. Straub-Bruce, BS Ed, RDH, Vermont: Healing Arts Press, 2014.

Cough

- **Elderberry Syrup (**)**

  Keep a 16 oz bottle on hand.

  Boosts immunity and shortens the duration of cold, cough, and flu.

- **Eucalyptus Essential Oil Steam**

  Keep a 1 oz bottle on hand.

  Use for steaming to reduce coughing and mucus. Steam alongside the antiviral tincture (**) and the Elderberry syrup (**).

Flu

- **Elderberry Syrup (**)**

  Keep one 16 oz bottle on hand.

  You will need to keep one cup of dried elderberries, one cup of honey, one cinnamon stick, one inch of fresh Ginger, and three clove buds on hand to make this recipe.

  Review the recipe for the ingredients and make one batch of syrup every season. Boosts immunity and shortens illness duration.

- **Peppermint Essential Oil Steam**

  Keep 1 oz on hand.

  It opens the lungs and helps clear congestion.

- **Antiviral Tincture (**)**

  Keep four two-ounce bottles on hand.

  They will last six months to a year, depending on your family size. See Chapter 7 for the exact amounts of herbal substances needed; the list is lengthy. The antiviral tincture clears chest congestion reduces fever and body aches. Use the tincture at the chronic dose level if you feel a cough developing suddenly.

- **Oregano essential oil**

  For steam inhalation to ease congestion.

Add a few drops of oregano essential oil to a bowl of steaming water. Lean over the bowl, covering your head with a towel, and inhale the steam to ease congestion and respiratory discomfort during cold, cough, and flu.

- **Thyme Tea**

  For respiratory support

  Keep dried thyme leaves on hand.

  Steep 1-2 teaspoons of dried thyme leaves in a cup of hot water for 10-15 minutes. Strain the tea and drink it to support respiratory health and boost the immune system. Thyme tea can be beneficial for middle-aged and senior individuals, especially during colder months.

Combination Cold, Cough, Flu

- **Peppermint Oil Steam**

  Keep a 1 oz bottle on hand for the whole family.

  Start steaming three times daily with **only one drop when the sniffles begin. Peppermint is powerful and can cause a burn if you get too close to the steam.**

- **Mullein (or Yarrow)**

  Keep 4 oz of either herb, or both, on hand.

  Yarrow and Mullein have similar qualities and are the same strength. Make the tea for a child at the first sign of a cough. It is safe for a child to take Mullein tea and Elderberry syrup. Even if a child does not have the flu, the Elderberry will boost immunity and shorten the duration of the cough.

- **Elderberry Syrup (**)**

  Keep 16 oz on hand each season for a family of four.

  The syrup will be your first line of defense for cold, cough, and flu. It is probably one of the top three most important things to have on hand. It only lasts about eight weeks if refrigerated.

- **The Facial Steam Thyme (with Mint and Oregano)**

  Inhalation can help alleviate congestion and minimize coughing.

  1. Bring a pot or tea kettle with about 4 cups of water to a boil.
  2. Place 3 tablespoons of Thyme in a large pot and pour the boiling water over them. Alternatively, you can mix Thyme with Mint and Oregano.
  3. Position your head over the pot, ensuring the steam is rising.
  4. Cover your head with a towel, creating a seal to trap the steam.
  5. Inhale the steam slowly and deeply for 5-8 minutes.

- **Basil Tea with Honey and Lemon**

  For relieving cold symptoms.

  Keep 1 oz of dried basil leaves and 8 oz of water on hand.

  Prepare the basil tea by steeping the dried basil leaves in hot water and sweeten with honey and lemon as desired. You will need 1 oz of dried basil leaves to make the tea.

Stomach Ache

- **Chamomile Flowers Tea/ Mint/ Oregano**

  Keep 4 oz of Chamomile/ Mint/ Oregano aerial parts on hand to calm the stomachache of a child or adult.

  This is a natural remedy to help with relaxation and sleep, calm the stomach, help against digestive spasms and internal colics.

- **Marshmallow Root Tea**

  For soothing an upset stomach

  Keep 1 tablespoon of dried marshmallow root and 1 cup of water on hand.

  To make marshmallow root tea, add the dried marshmallow root to a cup of boiling water. Let it steep for about 10 minutes, then strain the tea. Drink the marshmallow root tea to soothe digestive distress and alleviate an upset stomach.

Ear Ache

- **Mullein Ear Oil (Safe for Children)**

For ear infections

Keep 1 oz of the oil on hand.

You will only need 2 oz of dried Mullein flowers to make the ear oil. So, keep 2 oz of dried Mullein flowers on hand. The oil will last for two years if kept in the dark.

How its done:

1. Simmer two teaspoons of mullein flowers in ¼ cup olive oil for 20 minutes.
2. Strain into a glass vessel, then pour into a dropper bottle.
3. Let it cool.
4. Put one drop into the ear canal gently and massage the bony bump behind the ear to allow the oil to settle.
5. Lay on the opposite side and put in the second drop. Massage the back of that ear for a minute or so.
6. Two drops, three times daily, especially before bed, will help clear an ear infection.

Headache

- **Lemon Balm Tea**

Keep 4 oz of dried aerial parts on hand

- **Lavender Steam**

For headache relief.

Keep 1 oz of dried lavender flowers on hand.

Prepare the lavender steam by placing the dried lavender flowers in a small pouch or sachet. Inhale the soothing aroma of the lavender to help alleviate headaches. You will need 1 oz of dried lavender flowers.

Worms and Parasites

- **Mugwort Tincture**

  Keep 4 oz Mugwort aerial parts on hand (along with 8 oz of the alcohol of your choice to make the tincture)

  How it's done:

  Simple Mugwort Tincture for Worms and Parasites

  Follow the simpling method:

  1. Place four ounces of Mugwort in a clean glass jar.

  2. Cover with the alcohol of your choice, at least 60 proof.

  3. Let the herbs extract for twenty-one days.

  4. Strain the mixture, store it in a glass jar in a cool, dark place.

  For an acute situation, take the tincture every three hours for three days to expel the parasites. A tip: you can take hexane-free castor oil capsules to remove parasites and worms in addition to this tincture.

  Mugwort is a strong herb. The dosage will depend on how severe the condition is. Try the chronic dose and then increase it to four times a day if needed.

  Make four two-ounce tincture bottles to last a small family for up to two years. However, the tincture will store for several years.

- **Calendula Salve**

  For skin irritation and healing wounds

  Keep 2 oz of dried calendula flowers and 4 oz of carrier oil (such as olive oil) on hand.

  You will need 2 oz of dried calendula flowers to make the salve.

8.3 Immunity

We all need to pay careful attention to boosting immunity whenever possible. The very best remedy is prevention itself! It is vital to consume substances regularly that boost our immunity to have reserves for unforeseen circumstances.

Generally speaking, one ounce of an herb will last a child a week. Three to four ounces a week of most herbs is suitable for an adult.

Take one of the following depending on what is best for you and your family. You can combine the cookies or lozenges with any tea for daily support — just pay attention to the different dosage requirements for adults and children.

- **Rose Hips Tea**

  Keep 4 oz on hand.

- **Echinacea Tea**

  Keep 8 oz of Echinacea leaves on hand.

  Take the tea daily for up to three months.

- **Elderberry Syrup (**)**

  Keep 16 oz on hand for two adults and two children.

  Elderberry syrup can be combined with any tea, plus the throat lozenges or cookies as a sort of wellness package.

- **Echinacea/Ginger/Lemon First Aid Tonic**

  For increasing immunity (prepare two quarts weekly)

  Keep on hand 4 oz of Echinacea, three inches of Ginger, 1 lemon and honey to taste.

  1. Prepare one tablespoon of grated Ginger

  2. Measure 1 tablespoon of Echinacea

  3. Cut one lemon into quarters

  4. Set aside ¼ cup of honey

Decoct the ginger root in a quart of boiling water for twenty minutes. Add the echinacea and let it infuse for another 15 minutes.

Strain the mixture into a bowl. Add the juice of one lemon.

Add ¼ cup of honey (or sweeten to your taste).

Store in a glass container in the refrigerator for up to five days.

- **Immune-boosting cookies made with Echinacea**

  Good to have a batch on hand.

The cookies last for a couple of weeks if stored in an airtight container. One a day for prevention is enough.

How it's done:

Mixing powdered herbs into a cookie is a great way to distribute tasty preventative medicine or heal an already ill child.

1. Grind the dried fruits of your choice in a food processor or grinder.
2. Stir in coconut.
3. Mix in some peanut butter or another nut butter until you can roll the cookies into balls.
4. Measure how many cookies your batch will make.
5. Measure the amount of powdered herb your child will need in one cookie using the dosage measurements provided.
6. Measure the herb powder and mix it into the cookie dough.
7. Roll the cookies and serve.

Herbal powder options include Echinacea, Nettle, Yarrow, Mullein, or Mint. One or two cookies a day, in addition to tea dosages, makes healing more fun.

Please note: Onions and garlic are excellent immune boosters. Cook with them whenever possible. Both onions and garlic are blood pressure and blood sugar-stabilizing foods.

8.4   Skin Issues and Allergies

The following recipes are for oil extractions. Flowers and leaves are extracted and stored without cooking. Roots and heavier mediums are slow-cooked overnight.

- **Plantain Oil Extraction**

  For mild skin issues and itching

  1. In a quart-sized jar, place 1 cup of your dried plantain or two cups of fresh plantain.

  2. Cover the herb entirely with whatever oil you choose (Olive, almond, avocado, and apricot are good choices.)

  3. Cover the jar with a lid.

  4. Store in a cool, dark place for thirty to forty days. It takes a long time for oil extractions to complete.

  5. Shake the jar a couple of times a week to mix your ingredients.

  6. After the extraction is finished, strain the oil into a strainer lined with cheesecloth that sits over a bowl.

  7. After the oil drips through the cloth, gather the edges of the cloth. Twist and squeeze all of the oil out into the bowl.

  8. Pour the finished extraction into a glass jar.

  9. Store in a cool, dark place. Oleolites have a fair degree of shelf stability and will last for a couple of years when stored properly.

- **Plantain Poultice**

  For wounds, burns, and skin issues

  A Plantain poultice is a very powerful healer of skin tissue, and extracts toxins and infections from the skin. It has the power to reach beneath the subdermal layers. The herb is remarkable!

1. Gather ½ cup of dried leaves or 1 cup of fresh leaves. Macerate them with ¼ cup water. Add more if needed to make a paste.

2. Spread the paste on the affected area.

3. Cover with a 12" by 12 " clean cotton cloth (a sturdy paper towel is also fine).

4. Let the poultice work for 20 minutes to a half hour.

You can reuse this twice. then make a fresh batch. Repeat the process two to three times daily.

- **Anti-Allergen Tea with Nettle and Goldenrod**

Take this tea for allergies.

Adjust the dose for children. As the allergies subside, you can stop taking the tea.

If you know allergy season is coming, you can take this tea preventatively two weeks before your allergies usually start. Increasing your vitamin C intake at the same time by 500mg daily will also help.

1. Boil one quart of water.

2. Add one heaping teaspoon of dried Nettle.

3. Add one heaping teaspoon of dried Goldenrod.

4. Infuse for 15 minutes.

5. Strain into a clean glass vessel.

6. Drink three cups, morning, afternoon, and evening. Most teas store for three to four days.

8.5   Kidney Stone Prevention and Urinary Tract Infection

- **Horsetail Uva Ursi Tea**

    Keep 4 oz of Horsetail aerial parts and 4 oz of Uva Ursi on hand. (Uva Ursi is not otherwise mentioned in this book)

    Combine equal parts of these herbs to make this tea for two weeks. Then take a break for one week and resume if problems persist. Additionally, for urinary tract infections, you can take ¼ cup of cranberry juice three times daily to clean the walls of the urinary system.

    How its done:

    Take this tea for urinary tract infections. The horsetail is soothing, while Uva Ursi is highly astringent. It also helps to alternate this tea with ¼ cup of unsweetened cranberry juice throughout the day. Take this tea for three days. See a practitioner if your symptoms do not improve.

    1. Boil one quart of water.

    2. Add one heaping teaspoon of dried aerial Horsetail parts.

    3. Add one heaping teaspoon of dried Uva Ursi.

    4. Infuse for 15 minutes.

    5. Strain into a clean glass vessel.

    Drink three cups, morning, afternoon, and evening Most teas are store for three to four days.

8.6 Hypertension, Anemia and Blood Sugar Stabilization

Hypertension and Blood Sugar Stabilization

- **Ginger Root tea**

  Keep a small cluster or several inches of Ginger root on hand.

  Take three cups of tea daily for mild hypertension and blood sugar control. You can have either one condition or the other, or both. Ginger is an excellent way to address either issue, plus it will detoxify the blood and aid digestion. Ginger is a perfect remedy for aging in general.

- **Blackberry Soup**

  For reducing fatigue, gaining strength, and blood sugar stabilization

  1. Place one and ½ cups of blackberries in a small pot.

  2. Add ⅓ teaspoon cinnamon.

  3. Simmer for ten minutes and mash the berries with a potato masher.

  Cool and consume, just like soup. If you have the soup in the evening, it will help stabilize blood sugar levels throughout the night and reduce cravings the following day. One bowl of the soup long-term will help support adrenal function.

Anemia

- **Nettle/Red Clover Tea**

  Keep 4 oz on hand.

- **Red Clover**

  Keep 4 oz on hand.

  You will combine equal parts to make the Nettle/Red Clover tea. You can take this long-term safely. It is also an excellent nutritional and immune-boosting tonic.

- **Tea for Anemia and Fatty Liver (Red Clover Flowers/Yellow Dock Root)**

  Take this tea for anemia. It also facilitates weight loss.

  Drink plenty of water while taking this tea.

  1. Boil one quart of water.

  2. Add one heaping teaspoon of Yellow Dock root.

  3. Decoct for 20 minutes (on simmer).

  4. Add one heaping teaspoon of Red Clover flowers.

  5. Turn off the burner and infuse for 15 minutes.

  6. Strain into a clean glass vessel.

  Drink three cups morning in the afternoon, and evening Most teas are store for three to four days.

8.7   Energy and Concentration

The following remedies are arranged from the least strong to the strongest. Start with the first and move down the list progressively. However, do not take all the remedies at the same time! It will be too stimulating.

If you have gathered your herbs as directed up to this point, you will have the supplies needed for the following remedies.

- **Peppermint Steam** — Steam three times daily

  or

- **Echinacea/Ginger/Lemon Tonic** — Take three cups daily.

  Refer to the recipe for the portions. you will need to make a few quarts per week so plan accordingly.

  or

- **Ginseng Tea** — Take two cups daily, in the morning and afternoon.

  Keep 4 oz of dried American Ginseng root on hand.

Alternatively, you can make a vegetable soup and add **one ounce of Ginseng** to the soup as you boil it. Ensure that the Ginseng root is simmering in the soup for ½ hour. One or two bowls a day is a mild remedy that the whole family can consume.

Consuming the soup and steaming with mint oil are fine to do at separate times of the day. Both are gentle remedies and work well together.

8.8   Weight Loss and Detoxification

These weight loss remedies are meant to address congestion in the liver, break up fat cells, flush them out of the system, and tone the tissues to extract toxins.

- **Lemon/Ginger Echinacea Tonic**

  Keep a small cluster of Ginger, five lemons, and 4 oz Echinacea on hand. It will last you several days if you make a quart per day.

  For weight loss, take 3 cups daily. It is a wonderful immune-boosting remedy and very warming for those who get cold quickly.

- **Nettle/Rose Hips Tea**

  Keep 4 oz of Nettle and 4 oz of Rose Hips on hand.

  The tea will last you about two weeks if you take three cups daily. Nettle/Rose Hips tea is highly nutritious and also immune-boosting. It is a reliable remedy for both weight loss and daily immunity- and a bit stronger than the tonic above. Take three cups daily. It is not as warming as the Echinacea/Lemon/Ginger tonic due to the absence of Ginger.

- **Echinacea Tea**

  For detoxification, fatigue, and weight loss.

  Read the Materia Medica section on this herb. Echinacea works by clearing stagnation in the lymphatic system, blood, and liver. When stagnation is cleared it means that detoxification is the result. Detoxification often creates fatigue. It takes energy to move toxins out of the body. Please drink extra water when taking this herb.

1. Boil one quart of water.

2. Add three teaspoons of dried Echinacea leaves and flowers.

3. Infuse the herbs for 15 minutes.

4. Strain into a clean glass vessel

Drink three cups, morning, afternoon, and evening Most teas store for three to four days.

- **Daily Nutritive Tea**

  For weight loss (Nettle/Rose Hips)

  Take this tea for weight loss. It clears stagnation in the liver, nourishes all cells, and has an astringent quality. Astringents, typically sour sub- stances, break down and release fat cells from the body.

  1. Boil one quart of water.

  2. Add one heaping teaspoon of dried Nettle leaves.

  3. Add one heaping teaspoon of dried Rose Hips.

  4. Infuse for 15 minutes.

  5. Strain into a clean glass vessel.

  Drink three cups, morning, afternoon, and evening. Most teas store for three to four days.

- **Basil-infused water**

  Refreshing and detoxifying drink

  The advantages of basil-infused water include a refreshing taste, detoxifying properties, and potential support for weight loss, making it a healthy and flavorful beverage.

  Prepare the basil-infused water by adding the fresh basil leaves to a pitcher of water. Cutting or chopping the leaves helps to release the aromatic oils and compounds present in the leaves, which enhances the flavor and medicinal properties of the infusion. Let the mixture sit in the refrigerator for at least 4 hours to allow the flavors to infuse. Drink the basil-infused water as a refreshing and detoxifying beverage to support weight loss and promote detoxification. You will need 1 cup of fresh basil leaves to make the infused water.

- Parsley-infused water as a natural diuretic and detoxifying drink

Prepare parsley-infused water by steeping fresh parsley leaves in a glass of water for a few hours. Drink the infused water to promote diuresis and support detoxification

8.9   Remedies for Digestive Distress

- **Chamomile Tea**

Children and Adults for Digestive Distress (**)

Take this tea for depression or mild relaxation. Chamomile tea is also used for mild colds and sore throats.

- **Anti-Diarrhea Bath for Children (Blackberry Leaves)**

Take this bath instead of a dose of the blackberry tea to help control diarrhea.

1. Boil three quarts of water.
2. Add three heaping tablespoons of dried blackberry leaves.
3. Infuse for 20 minutes.
4. Strain into a clean glass vessel.
5. Run a hot bath.
6. Pour the concentrated tea into a shallow bath.
7. Let the child sit in the tub as usual. The tea will absorb into the skin.

- **Lemon Balm Tea**

For anxiety, digestion, mild colds with children or adults.

Take this tea for stomach aches, anxiety, mild cold, cough, and sore throat.

1. Boil one quart of water

2. Add three teaspoons of dried aerial Lemon Balm parts.

3. Infuse for 15 minutes.

4. Strain into a clean glass vessel.

5. Drink three cups, morning, afternoon, and evening. Adjust the dose for children.

Most teas store for three to four days

8.10 Memory Issues

- **Rosemary Hair Oil**

  For Memory, Energy, and Beautiful Hair

  Keep 4 oz of the oil extraction on hand.

  To make the extraction you will need 4 oz of the leaves and 4 oz of olive oil. Apply one to two times daily to the scalp and massage the oil into your head thoroughly.

  How it's done:

  o One cup of olive oil.

  o One cup of dried Rosemary leaves or 1 ½ fresh Rosemary leaves.

  Place the oil in a quart-sized glass jar. Sink the pot into three inches of water in a crockpot. Cover the crockpot and let the mixture cook overnight.

  Cool, and then strain in the morning into a clean glass jar. Store in a cool, dark, dry place. Take about a nickel-sized amount of oil and rub it on your palms. Thoroughly massage it into your scalp. It increases circulation to the scalp and restores both memory, stimulants cognition, and fortifies hair as well.

8.11 Anxiety, Insomnia, Fatigue and Depression

Anxiety

Passionflower tincture, lemon balm, chamomile, Lavender and California poppy tea are all known for their calming properties and potential to help reduce anxiety.

Lavender is well-known for its calming and relaxing properties, making it effective for reducing anxiety and promoting better sleep.

Passionflower is well-regarded for its anxiolytic effects and is commonly used to promote relaxation and ease anxiety symptoms. Lemon balm and chamomile are also known for their calming properties and have been traditionally used to soothe nerves and reduce anxiety. California poppy tea is known for its gentle sedative effects and may help promote relaxation.

Some people may find passionflower tincture more effective, while others may prefer lemon balm, chamomile, or California poppy tea. Additionally, combining certain herbs in a blend may provide synergistic effects, enhancing their overall calming properties.

Conscious or subconscious anxiety is often the cause of insomnia and stress.

- **Passionflower Tincture for Calming Anxiety:**
  1. Prepare a passionflower tincture by filling a glass jar with dried passionflower aerial parts and covering them with alcohol or glycerin.
  2. Let the mixture sit for 4-6 weeks, shaking occasionally.
  3. Strain the tincture and keep it in a dropper bottle.
  4. Administer a few drops under the tongue to calm anxiety and stress-related first aid situations.

- **California Poppy Remedy for Adult Anxiety**

  Keep 4 oz on hand.

It is a strong sedative and will work for both anxiety and insomnia.

- o Tea: Take two to three cups of tea daily.
- o Tincture (receipt below): Take 1" or one dropper full two to three times daily for anxiety or insomnia.
1. Gather one cup of flowers and seeds.
2. Place in a clean glass jar.
3. Cover with alcohol.
4. Let the mixture sit for twenty-one days.
5. Strain the mixture into a clean glass jar or two-ounce dropper bottles.
6. Store in a cool dark place.

The tea and the tincture are also recommended if you have problems with pain at night that keep you awake.

- **Chamomile Tea (**)**

Keep 4 oz on hand.

Brew chamomile tea using dried flowers and hot water. Drink it throughout the day to promote relaxation and soothe anxiety.

- **Lemon Balm Tea**

Keep 4 oz on hand.

Children or Adults For anxiety, digestion, mild colds

Take this tea for stomach aches, anxiety, mild cold, cough, and sore throat.

1. Boil one quart of water.
2. Add three teaspoons of dried aerial Lemon Balm parts.
3. Infuse for 15 minutes.
4. Strain into a clean glass vessel.
5. Drink three cups, morning, afternoon, and evening. Adjust the dose for children.

Most teas store for three to four days

Use lemon Balm Infused Oil (**) or as a Tincture:

Apply the oil topically or take a few drops of the tincture in water to alleviate anxiety.

Insomnia:

Most of the suggestions for insomnia will apply to anxiety as well. However, just take one tea at a time.

For **insomnia,** you may want to start your tea consumption later in the morning so that your last dose of tea is an hour before you go to sleep. Sedatives relax the nervous system while nervines tone the nervous system. California Poppy contains both actions but there are also other herbs that help with insomnia.

- **Lemon Balm Tea, Chamomile Tea** are mild remedies for anxiety.
- Keep 4 oz of either herb on hand.
- **California Poppy Tea**
- Either herb is a mild to medium-strength remedy for anxiety.
- Keep 4 oz of either herb on hand.
- **Rose Massage Oil and Rose Tea** will help with depression.
- Keep 4 oz of the extracted oil on hand.
- **Mint Tea** is a mild stimulant for depression and can provide temporary relief.
- Keep 4 oz of Peppermint or Spearmint leaves on hand.
- Most Mint leaves have very similar qualities.

Sleep / Fatigue

- Valerian tincture for addressing insomnia or sleep disturbances affecting sexual health.
- Take a few drops of valerian tincture orally to address insomnia or sleep disturbances that may affect sexual health. Valeri-

an's calming properties can contribute to better sleep and overall well-being in the context of sexual and reproductive health.

- Ginseng/ Dried Blackberry Tincture (for erectile dysfunction, strength, endurance)

- Review the recipe for your supplies and keep **two two-ounce dropper bottles** on hand.

- This formula is for invigoration and combatting long-term fatigue.

Also review the Insomnia section above and follow those guidelines.

Depression:

Best known to work for its benefits in managing depression is St. John's Wort. It has mood-enhancing properties and is often used as a natural remedy for mild to moderate depression.

- **St. John's Wort Infused Oil (**)**

It can be used topically for massage or as a soothing oil for skin conditions. It may also be used in aromatherapy diffusers for its mood-enhancing properties.

- **St. John's Wort Tincture**

How it's done:

1. Take dried St. John's Wort flowers (about 1 oz) and high-proof alcohol (such as vodka or brandy) – enough to cover the dried flowers.

2. Place the dried St. John's Wort flowers in a clean, dry glass jar.

3. Pour the alcohol over the flowers until they are fully covered.

4. Close the jar tightly and store it in a cool, dark place for about 4-6 weeks. Shake the jar gently every few days to mix the ingredients.

5. After the tincture has infused, strain the liquid using a fine mesh strainer or cheesecloth into a clean, dark glass dropper bottle.

UNLOCK THE SECRETS OF PLANT MEDICINE AT HOME

Store the St. John's Wort tincture in a cool, dark place. The recommended dosage is usually a few drops in water or tea, taken up to three times a day.

- **Passionflower (*Passiflora incarnata*)**

  Passionflower has natural sedative and anxiolytic (anxiety-reducing) effects, making it effective for both anxiety and insomnia.

Lethargy and Lack of Concentration

- **Peppermint Essential Oil Steam**

  Keep 1 oz on hand for steaming.

  Again, remember to steam with one drop only and keep the face at least a foot above the steam while you close your eyes.

8.12 Remedies for Beauty

Beauty and wellness depend on proper nutrition, adequate sleep, healthy family life, social connections, and other aspects. However, herbs can certainly help, and it is worth making your beauty products with ingredients that you can trust.

This book presents a weekly nighttime regime:

1. Steam the pores open with the Rose petal face steam.

2. Apply the Nettle Green Clay face mask after patting the face dry from steaming.

3. Ending with a thin application of the Rose massage oil. Repeat once weekly. The routine pampers and restores.

How it's done:

- **Rose Petals**

  Keep 6 oz on hand.

  You will use this to make the Rose massage oil and also for the Rose petal/Sage face steam.

Place one teaspoon each of Rose petals and Sage in a small pot of hot steaming water. Make a tent over your head with a hand towel and put your face one foot above the pot. Allow the vapors to open your pores for a few minutes.

After steaming, dry the skin and apply the Nettle face pack below.

- **Nettle Face Mask**

Keep 2 oz on hand

How it's done:

Nettle Face Mask (Green face mask to detoxify and regenerate)

1. Put one teaspoon of Nettle powder in a small bowl.
2. Add four teaspoons of French Green Clay.
3. Add three drops of lavender essential oil.
4. Mix the ingredients into a paste.

Take one teaspoon of the paste and spread it over your face without coming too close to the eyes. Let it dry until it begins to crack. Take a hot steaming washcloth, ring it out and remove your mask. Repeat until you remove the mask. Proceed with your usual routine.

Overnight, apply some of the Rose massage oil as a deep emollient.

- **Green Clay**

Keep 2 oz on hand.

Another possibility is:

- **Lavender Water** as a toner for the skin
    1. Take 1/4 cup of dried lavender flowers and 1 cup of distilled water.
    2. Place the dried lavender flowers in a heat-resistant bowl and pour boiling distilled water over them.
    3. Cover the bowl and let it steep for about 15 minutes.

4. Strain the liquid and let it cool.

5. Transfer the lavender water to a clean, airtight container and store it in the refrigerator.

Use lavender water as a toner for the skin to enhance beauty and refresh your complexion. You will need 1/4 cup of dried lavender flowers to make the lavender water.

8.13 Sexual and Reproductive Health

At this point in your herbal shopping, you will have acquired all of the herbs needed for this section.

Sexual health improves through lifestyle factors, especially sleep. The second factor to address is underlying issues such as anxiety and depression. Another factor that increases sexual vitality and confidence is weight loss. Think carefully about whether any of these issues apply to you. When reviewing the following section, choose the most appropriate tea for you. Four ounces of your chosen ingredient will be enough for the standard dose while consuming the tea for two weeks.

The remedies proceed from number one to number four by order of strength. Review the formulas for anxiety, depression, and insomnia very carefully. If you decide to make these formulas, go back and look at the Materia Medica. If you are uncertain about what you need, follow the guidance of a practitioner.

The remedies against anxiety, stress, insomnia, Fatigue, and Depression have been added to a separate chapter. Please consult Chapter 8.10 to address these issues.

Sexual Vitality and Reproductive Health

- **Passionflower Tea or Tincture**

  For Stress-Related Reproductive Issues

  Prepare passionflower tea by steeping dried passionflower aerial parts in hot water for 10-15 minutes. Strain the tea and drink it or use a passionflower tincture to manage stress-related reproductive issues.

- **Ginseng Tea**

  For stamina and to increase libido

  1. Boil one quart of water.
  2. Add one tablespoon of Ginseng root.
  3. Decoct the root for 20 minutes.
  4. Strain the decoction into a clean glass vessel.
  5. Drink only two cups, morning and afternoon. Ginseng is too stimulating to take in the late afternoon and evening.

  Most teas store for three to four days. Ginseng tea will increase both stamina and libido. Alternatively, you can decoct two tablespoons of the root, tied in cheesecloth in a typical vegetable soup. A milder dose of Ginseng along with vegetables and broth is excellent preventative medicine for the whole family!

Sexual Tonic for Women

- **Rose/Lemon Balm/ Chamomile/Mint**

  This recipe is a tonic nervine and mood-enhancing tea. It works well when combined with the Rose massage oil. Remember that sexual desire is often enhanced by stress reduction, balancing lifestyle issues, and increasing self-esteem.

  1. Boil two quarts of water.
  2. Add 1/2 tablespoon each dried Rose, Lemon Balm, and Chamomile.
  3. Add one teaspoon of Mint
  4. Infuse for 15 minutes
  5. Strain into a clean glass vessel
  6. Drink three cups, morning, afternoon, and evening Most teas store for three to four days.

Take a break periodically from this tonic for four days and then resume for long-term use.

For erectile dysfunction, strength, endurance

- **Ginseng/ Dried Blackberry Tincture**

  Review the recipe for your supplies and keep two two-ounce dropper bottles on hand.

  This formula is for invigoration and combatting long-term fatigue.

  1. Place equal parts, ¼ cup each of Ginseng and dried Blackberries in a quart jar.

  2. Use the simpling method and cover with the alcohol of your choice.

  Let the tincture extract for twenty-one days. Strain it and pour it into a glass jar or 2-ounce dropper bottle.

  Take 1" or one dropper full three times daily, morning, afternoon, and evening.

Menstruation and Hormone Balance

- **Menstrual Formula for Teens and Adults**

  Black Cohosh and Dried Blackberry Tincture

  This tincture is commonly used for women's health issues, particularly to support menstrual health. Additionally, Black Cohosh contains compounds that are thought to have estrogen-like effects, which may help to alleviate hormonal imbalances in menopausal and perimenopausal women.

  1. Place equal parts, ¼ cup each of Black Cohosh and dried Blackberries in a quart jar.

  2. Use the simpling method and cover with the alcohol of your choice.

3. Let the tincture extract for twenty-one days. Strain it and pour it into a glass jar or two-ounce dropper bottles.

4. Take 1" or one dropper full three times daily, morning, afternoon, and evening.

For Relaxation and Romance

- **Rose Massage Oil**

    1. In a quart-sized jar, place 1 cup Rose petals.

    2. Cover the petals entirely with whatever oil you choose (olive, almond, avocado, apricot are good choices)

    3. Cover the jar with a lid.

    4. Store in a cool, dark place for thirty to forty days. It takes a long time for oil extractions to complete.

    5. Shake the jar a couple of times a week to mix your ingredients.

    6. After the extraction is finished, strain the oil into a strainer lined with cheesecloth that sits over a bowl.

    7. After the oil drips through the cloth, gather the edges of the cloth. Twist and squeeze all of the oil out into the bowl.

    8. Pour the finished extraction into a glass jar.

    9. Store in a cool, dark place. Oleolites have a fair degree of shelf stability and will last for a couple of years when stored properly.

9   Overview List of Conditions and Corresponding Healing Herbs

The following table provides a list of herbal uses at a glance for quick reference. Notice that you can sometimes substitute one herb for another.

Ailment	symptom	Herbal aids					
Abdominal Cramping		Black Co-hosh	Chamomile	Meadow-sweet	Sage	Oregano	
Allergies		Goldenrod	Nettles				
Anemia		Blackberries	Nettles	Red Clover	Yellow Dock		
Ankles, swollen		Arnica	Echinacea	Rose Hips			
Anxiety		Chamomile	California Poppy	Lavender	Lemon Balm	Passion-flower	Valerian
Arthritis		Arnica	Comfrey	Elderberry	Wild Ginger	Meadow-sweet	
Beauty	skin	Rose	Plantain				

Ailment	symptom	Herbal aids					
Bladder Infection	hair	Rosemary	Nettles				
		Marshmallow					
Blood Pressure	high	Wild Ginger	Passionflower	Yarrow			
	low	Rosemary	Rosemary				
	cardiotonic	Milkweed	Milkweed				
Bones	aching	Boneset	Boneset				
	injured	Arnica	Comfrey				
Bowels		Chamomile	Mint				
Bronchial	congestion	Thyme	Boneset	Milkweed	Ginger	Mullein	Marshmallow
	dry cough	Elderberry	Ginger	Sage	Marshmallow		
	wet cough	Black Cohosh	Ginger	Milkweed	Sage	Mullein	
	cold chest	Ginger	Milkweed				
	hot chest	Mint					

UNLOCK THE SECRETS OF PLANT MEDICINE AT HOME

Ailment	symptom	Herbal aids							
Circulation		Ginger	Rosemary	Yarrow					
Constipation			Ginger						
Depression		St. John's Wort	Passion-flower	Basil (1)	Chamomile	Lemon Balm	Rose		
Diarrhea		Blackberry	Sage						
Diaper Rash		Mullein leaf	Plantain						
Digestion		'bitter' herb (2)	Basil	Thyme					
Earache		Mullein oil							
Emotional Challenges		California Poppy	Chamomile	Dandelion flr.	Lemon Balm	Rosemary	Sage	Rose	Lavender
Fatigue/Exhaustion		Blackberries	Rosemary	Sage	Lavender	Passion-flower			
Flu (antiviral)		Elderberry	Boneset	Ginger					

(1) Better known as a strong adaptogen is the basil species Tulsi/Holy Basil

(2) See herbal actions in Chapter 2.3. Bitter herbs are known for their ability to stimulate the digestive system, particularly the release of digestive hormones and bile flow. These herbs help improve appetite, promote digestion, and support liver function, making them beneficial for overall gut health.

Ailment	symptom	Herbal aids							
Fever		Basil	Boneset	Elderberry	Meadow-sweet	Yarrow			
Headaches		Basil	Lemon Balm	Mint	Sage	Lavender			
Ailment	Symptom	Herbal aids							
Hemor-rhoids		St. John's Wort oil	Plantain	Mugwort					
Immune boost		Elderberry	Ginger	Ginseng	Rose Hips				
Indigestion		Chamomile	Lemon Balm	Mint	Sage				
Inflamma-tion		Chamomile	Comfrey	Dandelion	Wild Ginger	Goldenrod	Lemon Balm	Meadow-sweet	Calendula
Insomnia		California Poppy	Chamomile	Lemon Balm	Valerian				
Kidney	infection	Milkweed	Thyme						
	adrenal fatigue	Blackberries	Ginseng	Rose Hips					
Lethargy/ lack of Con-centration		Ginseng	Mint	Rosemary	Sage				

Ailment	symptom	Herbal aids	Dandelion	Nettles	Oregano	Yellow Dock
Liver	congestion	Comfrey	Ginger	Milkweed	Mullein	Thyme
Lung	congestion	Boneset	Mullein	Thyme		
	inflammation	Boneset	Ginger	Mullein	Thyme	
	infection	Boneset				
Memory Loss		Rosemary				
Ailment	Symptom	Herbal aids				
Menstruation	regulation	Black Cohosh	Calendula	Yarrow	Parsley	
	hot flashes	Sage	Black Cohosh			
	night sweats	Sage	Nettles	Rose Hips		
	weight gain	Echinacea	Lemon Balm			
	depression	Mint	Rosemary			
Muscular	soreness	Arnica	Chamomile	Rosemary		
	spasms	Black Cohosh	Passionflower	Valerian		

Ailment	symptom	Herbal aids					
	inflammation	Arnica	Meadow-sweet				
Nausea		Wild Ginger	Oregano				
Parasites		Mugwort					
Poison Ivy		Plantain					
Rheumatism		Arnica	Meadow-sweet	Nettles			
Sinus Infections		Mint					
Sexual Health		Ginseng	Rose				
Stings		Plantain					
Throat (sore)		Elderberry	Ginger	Lemon Balm	Mint	Mullein	Rose Hips
Tooth Pain		Sage					
Varicose Veins		Ginger	Dock	Red Clover	Yarrow		
Vomiting	to prevent/stop	Mint	Oregano	Meadow-sweet			
	induce	Boneset					

Ailment	symptom	Herbal aids					
Weight Loss		Echinacea	Ginger	Nettles			
Worms		Mugwort					
Wounds		Comfrey (not open wounds)	Plantain	Yarrow (stop bleeding)	Milkweed	St. John's Wort	Oregano oil

10 Cultivating a Holistic Lifestyle with Plant Medicine

As we come to the end of this journey through the world of herbs and their incredible healing potential, I invite you to reflect on the countless ways you can incorporate these natural wonders into your daily life. From savoring herbal teas to creating personalized remedies, you now hold the keys to unlocking a harmonious and balanced lifestyle.

By growing some of the plants presented in this book yourself, you can deepen the power of herbs and their profound impact on your well-being. May this newfound knowledge empower you to address specific health concerns and curate your own herbal apothecary with confidence and purpose.

As you continue on your holistic herbal journey, remember that this is just the beginning. There is so much more to explore, and each discovery will deepen your understanding of the intricate relationship between nature and our well-being. Embrace complementary practices such as meditation, yoga, and self-care rituals to nurture not only your body but also your mind and spirit.

I hope this book has inspired you to view herbs as more than just remedies but as allies on your path to holistic wellness. May you cherish the connection you have formed with these magnificent plants and continue to embrace the wisdom they offer.

11   Sources

(1)   'Herbs for Healthy Aging: Natural Prescriptions for Vital Health', Vermont: Healing Arts Press, 2014.

(2)   American Herbalists Guild, Herbal Medicine F.A.Q.s | American Herbalists Guild, Seen: January 21, 2020

(3)   American Society for Clinical Oncology, Memorial Sloan Kettering, June 25, 2016. Seen on: Black Cohosh — The ASCO Post, (www.ascopost.com)

(4)   Apaydin EA, Maher AR, Shanman R, Booth MS, Miles JN, Sorbero ME, Hempel S. A systematic review of St. John's wort for major depressive disorder. Syst Rev. 2016 Sep 2;5(1):148. doi: 10.1186/s13643-016-0325-2. PMID: 27589952; PMCID: PMC5010734., see: *https://www.ncbi.nlm.nih.gov/pmc/articles/PMC5010734/*

(5)   Arsić I, Zugić A, Tadić V, Tasić-Kostov M, Mišić D, Primorac M, Runjaić-Antić D. Estimation of dermatological application of creams with St. John's Wort oil extracts. Molecules. 2011 Dec 28;17(1):275-94. doi: 10.3390/molecules17010275. PMID: 22205093; PMCID: PMC6268942., see: *https://pubmed.ncbi.nlm.nih.gov/22205093/*

(6)   Dawid-Pać R. Medicinal plants used in treatment of inflammatory skin diseases. Postepy Dermatol Alergol. 2013 Jun;30(3):170-7. doi: 10.5114/pdia.2013.35620. Epub 2013 Jun 2000., see *https://www.ncbi.nlm.nih.gov/pmc/articles/PMC3834722/*

(7)   Gallegos, Robert, "A Native American Traditional Healer Teaches About Self-Healing", June 18, 2017, Native American Traditional Healer teaching about self-healing — YouTube, Seen on February 20, 2022.

(8)   Gladstar, Rosemary "The Science and Art of Herbalism," Vermont: Sage Mountain Press, 2014.

(9) Green, Matthew, "The Native American Healer Reviving The History of Her Ancestors," Interview with Linda Black Elk, Minnesota Public Radio, December 31, 2018

(10) Hoffman, David FNIMH, AHG, "Herbs for Healthy Aging: Natural Prescriptions for Vibrant Health" Vermont: Healing Arts Press, 2014. (See: Sarsaparilla)

(11) Hoffman, David, FNIMH, AHG, "The Complete Illustrated Holistic Herbal: A Safe and Practical Guide to Making and Using Herbal Remedies", Australia: Element Books Limited, 1996.

(12) *https://extension.usu.edu/rangeplants/forbs-herbaceous/horsetail*

(13) J Vlachojannis, F Magora, S Chrubasik. July 25th, 2011 Jul, Willow species and aspirin: different mechanism of actions. Phytother Res: 1102-4. doi: 10.1002/ptr.3386. (*https://pubmed. ncbi.nlm.nih.gov/21226125/*)

(14) Jean M. Bokelmann, Medicinal Herbs in Primary Care, Elsevier, Passionflower: Pages 515-522, ISBN 9780323846769, 2022, *https:// www.sciencedirect.com/science/article/pii/B9780323846769000635*

(15) Koetter, U., Schrader, E., Käufeler, R. and Brattström, A. (2007), A randomized, double-blind, placebo-controlled, prospective clinical study to demonstrate clinical efficacy of a fixed valerian hops extract combination (Ze 91019) in patients suffering from non-organic sleep disorder. Phytother. Res., 21: 847-851. *https://doi.org/10.1002/ptr.2167*

(16) Kreiger, Diane, "USC Pharmacist Uncovers Healing Powers of Native Plants," USC Trojan Family, Winter 2014

(17) Mojay, Gabriel, "Aromatherapy for Healing the Spirit: Restoring Emotional and Mental Balance with Essential Oils", Vermont: Healing Arts Press, 1997.

(18) Muhammad Asif Hanif, Samir AlAdawi, Basil: A natural source of antioxidants and neutraceuticals in book: Natural Products and Their Active Compounds on Disease Prevention (pp.463-471), August 2012

UNLOCK THE SECRETS OF PLANT MEDICINE AT HOME

(19) Nafiseh Shokri Mashhadi, Reza Ghiasvand, Gholamreza Askari, Mitra Hariri, Leila Darvishi, and Mohammad Reza Mofid, "Anti-Oxidative and Anti-Inflammatory Effects of Ginger in Health and Physical Activity: Review of Current Evidence" International Journal of Preventive Medicine, 2013 Apr; 4(Suppl 1): S36–S42., Seen on: *https://www.ncbi.nlm.nih.gov/pmc/articles/PMC3665023/*, January 27, 2022

(20) Shaeffer, Elizabeth, "Dandelion, Pokeweed, and Coltsfoot: How the early settlers used plants for food, medicine and in their home," Dandelion, Addison-Wesley: Massachusetts, 1972

(21) Staiger C. Comfrey: a clinical overview. Phytother Res. 2012;26(10):1441-1448. doi:10.1002/ptr.4612, see: *https://www.ncbi.nlm.nih.gov/pmc/articles/PMC3491633/*

(22) Tierra, Michael, L.Ac. O.M.D., "The Way of Herbs," New York: Pocket Books, 1998.

(23) U.S. Department of Agriculture (USDA), FoodData Central Search Results: Thyme Fresh, April 2019. see: *https://fdc.nal.usda.gov/fdc-app.html#/food-details/173470/nutrients*

(24) USDA Forest Service, Boise, Heartleaf Arnica, Seen on: Boise National Forest — Nature & Science (usda.gov), Utah State University, *https://www.fs.usda.gov/detail/boise/learning/nature-science/?cid=fsed_009691*

(25) Yance, Donald R., C.N., MH, R.H. (AHG), "Adaptogens in Medical Herbalism" Vermont: Healing Arts Press, 2014.

(26) Zhang, Junhua, et al., "The Safety of Herbal Medicine: From Prejudice to Evidence" Evidence-Based Complementary and Alternative Medicine, Hindawi Publishing Corporation, Volume 2015 |Article ID 316706 | *https://doi.org/10.1155/2015/316706*

FREE GIFT TO OUR READERS
Cook with Medical Herbs and Plants

Integrate healing plants and herbs in your daily routine **Get 20 free recipes** on how you can use the herbs and plants presented in this book for cooking.

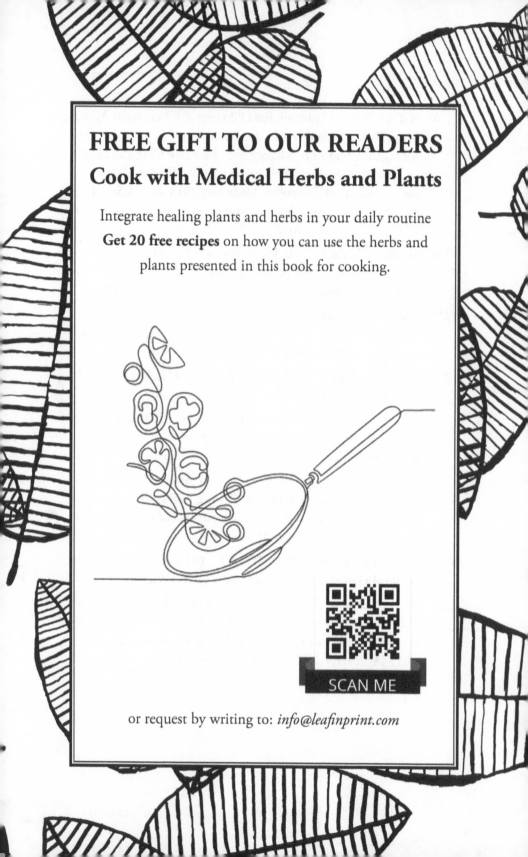

SCAN ME

or request by writing to: *info@leafinprint.com*

WITH SEASONAL HARVESTING CHART

FROM THE SAME PUBLISHER

Foraging Medicinal Herbs and Wild Edible Plants in the Great Lakes Region

Upper Midwest and Ontario - Identify, Harvest, Prepare and Store Wild Foods and Healing Herbs and Plants

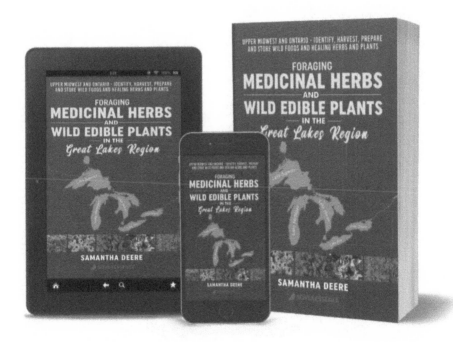

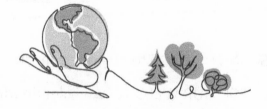

Version v1 – 9.2023